THE LOW BLOOD SUGAR
GOURMET COOKBOOK

THE LOW BLOOD SUGAR GOURMET COOKBOOK

by Sylvia G. L. Dannett
with Maureen McCabe

Foreword by A. B. Vivera, M.D.

DRAKE PUBLISHERS INC NEW YORK

Published in 1974 by
Drake Publishers Inc.
381 Park Avenue South
New York, New York 10016

© Sylvia G. L. Dannett with Maureen McCabe, 1974

Library of Congress Cataloging in Publication Data

Dannett, Sylvia G L   1909–
   The low blood sugar gourmet cookbook.
   1. Cookery for hypoglycemics.   I. McCabe, Maureen,
joint author.   II. Title.
RM221.H9D36   641.5′638   73–18182
ISBN 0–87749–599–8

Printed in the United States of America

Contents

Foreword by A. B. Vivera, M.D. vii

How I Discovered That I Had Low Blood Sugar
and Did Something About It—You Can, Too! 1

Condiments 5

A Note on Frying 6

For Your Sweet Tooth 6

Menus 7

 Breakfast 7

 Lunch 16

 Dinner 22

Appetizers and Snacks 33

Breads, Muffins and Biscuits 39

Soups 46

Salads 54

Eggs 63

Meats 66

Fish 93

Vegetables 104

Casseroles 118

Sauces, Dressings, Toppings and Garnishes 123

Desserts 132

Index 155

Foreword

H ypoglycemia, or simply stated, low blood sugar, is increasingly recognized as an important cause of a variety of unpleasant symptoms. Days which start out with a feeling of tiredness even after what seems hours of sleep or rest, chronic fatigue, nagging headaches, poor concentration, moments of weakness, clumsiness, depression, may all be manifestations of hypoglycemia. Except in the more severe forms, these symptoms may not be incapacitating, but are certainly debilitating enough to make life a matter of day-to-day existence without pleasure or joy—living becomes a chore.

Fortunately, the presence of hypoglycemia can be ascertained by a physician after a thorough examination and use of the proper laboratory procedures. Once established, treatment designed to correct the low blood sugar—a hypoglycemia diet with or without other medications—will be prescribed. Here, we are concerned mainly with the dietary aspect of the treatment.

The prime objective of all diets for hypoglycemia is the maintenance of a fairly uniform and adequate blood sugar level. This is achieved essentially by a diet high in proteins and low in carbohydrates and sugar content. Meals should be frequent, at least six times a day. Some of these may be in the form of snacks.

As with any diet, success depends not only on the patient's understanding of the basic necessary items, but that each meal will be attractive, appetizing and palatable. It is not sufficient to have merely a list of allowed or prohibited foods. Ease and simplicity in planning and preparation of such meals can contribute to the patients' interest and enthusiasm for their diet. In this way there is a greater chance that the patients not only will adopt the diet, but that they will be encouraged, as well, to change their food patterns by integrating their diet into their mode of living.

Mrs. Dannett and Mrs. McCabe in this book have eased the difficulties of nutritional planning. With their ingenuity and culinary expertise they have produced an amazing variety of recipes and menu ideas which are simple and practicable. Indeed they have rendered a great service not only to the hypoglycemia sufferers but to everyone, since a high-protein and low-carbohydrate-sugar diet, unless medically prohibited, is basically nutritionally desirable. Those who wish to reduce certainly will welcome the recommendations of the authors. Besides being low in calories and high in proteins and healthful the menus are appetizing and *satisfying*.

A. B. Vivera, M.D.

How I Discovered That I Had Low Blood Sugar and Did Something about It —You Can, Too!

T his discovery that I had a mild case of hypoglycemia forced me to alter the eating habits of a lifetime. That it came as a well-disguised blessing is an understatement. I, who finished a box of chocolates at one sitting at least twice monthly, ate three or four slices of coffee cake for breakfast several mornings a week, gorged on desserts like devil's food cake and chocolate soufflé, now had to come to grips with the fact that sugar, chocolate, coffee, cola drinks and ice cream were out of my gustatory bounds. How sad. So I thought.

Dissolved in self-pity, I mentally began listing many other delights I would henceforth be denied. No more corn on the cob for dinner every night in summer. No iced coffee, ice cream nor raspberry sherbet. No more delicious fresh limas and beets vinaigrette. No more nice low-calorie carbohydrate lunches such as half a melon with cottage cheese, a grilled cheese sandwich, or just a salad and a diet coke. What would become of my admired figure now that I had to eat six times a day? How could I avoid putting on weight?

Misery, of course, loves company, and I was pleased to discover that there were approximately 799,000 other people in the United States with low blood sugar. How good to know I had something in common with so many! I began to wonder what these others were doing about their diets and how they adjusted to such drastic changes in their eating habits. It would be nice, I thought, almost wistfully, if there were an HG club or if we had get-togethers like the weight-watchers to exchange ideas.

In the ensuing weeks I stumbled through a dietetic wilderness. The idea of eating six times a day was getting me down. Yet, fearful of dizziness, blackouts, and exhaustion and depression I forced myself to adhere to the foods prescribed. When I felt like nibbling I resorted to nuts, which I had ignored for years as being fattening and indigestible. Now I found the dry roasted peanuts or almonds delicious. After all, I told myself, they were

1

protein, and protein was good for me. I soon reached the high water mark of seven ounces of nuts in an evening while writing. My doctor told me this was equivalent to a pound of meat and too heavy a load for my stomach. The odd part of it was while eating more often and more substantially I had begun to lose weight. This is not uncommon, I discovered, in the early stages of the diet.

Unaccustomed to nutritional planning of this sort I carefully studied my doctor's dos and don'ts as well as his two breakfast menus; Carleton Fredericks' book *Low Blood Sugar* which presented a good consistent overall picture of the illness and was helpful on snacks; Doctor Clement G. Martin's *The Hidden Menace of Hypoglycemia* with its three sets of diets for low-blood-sugar patients, with drastic differences between them. Adelle Davis, who believes HG has become a major health problem in the United States, gave me further insight into the mineral and vitamin needs of our bodies and the importance of establishing proper eating habits. Later, in working out all-inclusive menus I profited by her knowledge and included whenever possible, green vegetables, yeast, wheat germ, and whole-grain bread—the latter primarily home-baked—in my menus. Articles —there weren't many—gave me little tidbits of information and brought me to the end of my research. I still hadn't received any long-range suggestions nor read recipes that would enhance my diet, and came to the conclusion that HG foods needed a little excitement. There was no cookbook available for low-blood-sugar patients, and the few menus offered were limited and tiresome. A gourmet cookbook with menus and recipes was needed and I decided to strike out for myself. Tackling the problem head-on, I determined to write a hypoglycemia gourmet cookbook, hoping to help all victims of this illness, not just myself. Through trial and error, I would be my own guinea pig. What enticing dishes I would create!

I had made a number of discoveries on my own that enabled me to form certain conclusions. If I ate a great deal of protein, I lost my craving for sweets. My own body and my doctor told me meat for breakfast at least four times a week was a must. I found early-morning depression or exhaustion soon disappeared. Friends of mine threw up their hands in horror at this suggestion which is, of course, ridiculous. Up at our fishing club we sometimes have fish for breakfast and ham, sausages, or bacon with eggs. Broiled, fresh-caught calico bass, or halibut, broiled or baked, hot or cold, for breakfast, are satisfying, fresh and delicate in taste, and energy-producing. While the idea of breakfasting on steak, hamburgers, veal and lamb chops may seem a bit hearty for those of you who are accustomed to a light, low-calorie breakfast, as it was to me, be brave, as I was. I'll admit I tried chicken first; it seemed such a nice, feminine dish. Feminine it may be, but it won't build up energy like a four-ounce shell steak or an inch-thick veal chop. I will admit, though, that it was months before I could face a steak at seven-thirty in the morning.

It wasn't an easy task I had set for myself. I started by dreaming up snacks first. My creations were well received by guests and fellow-sufferers. Thank heaven for cheese in all its varieties! Your taste buds can be titillated daily. Desserts, the second target of attack, were my particular *bête noir*. I emerged from a period of trial and error with results. Now when diabetic or weight-watching friends come to dinner they welcome my sugar- and fat-free concoctions, and don't miss the pies and cakes served to the other guests.

The suggested vegetables for the diet proved to be monotonous after awhile, even with variations in preparation. My doctor then told me about substitution. Forgo a slice of bread on certain days, he said, and eat the prohibited baked potato, carrots, winter squash or peas, and the like. This was great news, and offered me the opportunity of making my menus more varied.

Gradually I began to achieve a healthy balance in my diet. Adjusted to the change, I rather enjoyed my man-sized breakfasts. I stopped gorging on peanuts and discovered that it was better to take a handful or two of nuts after each meal. I stopped losing, went back to my original weight and have stayed there.

Suddenly I awakened to the fact that I was my old vigorous, energetic driving self. So sad about having hypoglycemia? Not any longer!

About this time I combined forces with Maureen McCabe, a top-notch cook and caterer. We experimented, we did research. I walked around carrying my stove in my brain, and started cooking literally and mentally. Maureen and I cooked and she baked, aware of the need for tasty starch-free, molasses-free, sugar-free, etc. breads and muffins. We shopped the health stores as well as out-of-the-way food stores. We planned menus for breakast, lunch and dinner. One meal led to another, and finally, one day we decided we had enough material for this book.

We hope you will follow our menus and then try our recipes.

How I Discovered That I Had Low Blood Sugar

Eat and enjoy the HG way. Remember, however, that your case may be more severe than mine. No two patients are alike. Leave out any ingredients like ordinary or seasoned salt, for example, if it is not on your diet. There are good salt substitutes. In fact, there are adequate substitutes for almost everything. You won't be hungry. You'll have new energy, remain slim and find that you enjoy life again.

Sylvia G. L. Dannett

Sugar-Free
Condiments and Flavorings
You Can Use
Plus Extracts to
Ask Your Doctor About
and
Recommended Salad Oils,
Peanut Butter, Other Provisions

Featherweight's Imitation Sugar-free Catsup ***

Featherweight's Sugar-free Chili Sauce ***

Tabasco

Dijon Mustard

All No-Cal Fruit Flavorings

Sherman's Low-Calorie Pancake Syrup (imitation maple) ***

Old-Fashioned Peanut Butter with salt ***

Elam's Peanut Butter without salt or sugar ***

Cottonseed *** or Safflower Oil

Mayo 7 ***

Artificial sweeteners we prefer: Twin Sugar packages; loose Sweet'N Low for cooking; Featherweight's Calorie-free Sweetening (no cyclamate) *** (3 drops approx. 1 tsp. sugar)

All Wagner's "Pure Extracts" such as rum, peppermint, lime, lemon, walnut and the like contain approximately 69 percent alcohol. A few drops go a long way, but better check with your doctor before using.

*** Buy in Health Food Store

A NOTE ON FRYING

When we say fried in this book, we mean to fry in a nonstick pan with just enough diet margarine to keep the food from sticking.

FOR YOUR SWEET TOOTH

Since sugar is out of your diet, it is well to know what you are using in the artificial line.

There are dozens of *packets* on the market. Each packet generally is equal in sweetness to 2 teaspoons of sugar.

There are dozens of *liquid* artificial sweeteners. Some prefer these for cooking. We rarely use any of them. For the liquid, the count is as follows: ⅛ of a teaspoon = 1 teaspoon of sugar. Usually a person uses 6 drops per serving of decaffeinated coffee or weak tea. Some like to use more. 1 tbsp. of liquid = ½ cup of sugar. The calories are negligible. There are shakers of powdered sweetener on the market. 2 shakes = approximately 1 tsp. of sugar and contain less than 10 mg. of saccharin.

There are also artificial sweeteners that come loose in a box. The loose form is essential for baking and some cooking. There is a tiny spoon in the box which you must use. The following are the quantities which equal an equivalent sweetness in terms of sugar:

$\frac{1}{10}$ tsp. of the powder = 1 tsp. of sugar
$\frac{1}{3}$ tsp. of the powder = 1 tbs. of sugar
1 tsp. of the powder = $\frac{1}{6}$ cup of sugar
3 tsp. of the powder = $\frac{1}{2}$ cup of sugar
6 tsp. of the powder = 1 cup of sugar

Menus

Top of the Morning

Breakfast is your most important meal. It can become your most interesting meal. We offer 39 suggestions for starting your day right. You'll feel satisfied and slim and will have done right by your low-blood-sugar condition. Don't be dismayed if there is an outcry about your man-sized breakfast. New Englanders have always believed in eating meat or fish for breakfast, and at all the fishing camps and our fishing club we have either fresh-caught fish, or ham, sausages or bacon with or without eggs. Think *meat* at breakfast time and enjoy yourself!

The menus given are to follow the pre-breakfast drink prescribed by many doctors for hypoglycemia patients.

4 ounces fresh grapefruit juice or unsweetened
canned juice
2 shirred eggs
1 slice toasted soy-oat bread ***
Diet or regular margarine
1 tbs. natural peanut butter ***
Decaffeinated coffee—fat-free or whole milk
Artificial sweetener

¼ cantaloupe
2 scrambled eggs with Cheddar cheese
1 slice whole-wheat toast
Diet or regular margarine, or butter
Decaffeinated coffee—fat-free or whole milk
Artificial sweetener

*** Buy in Health Food Store

1 veal chop weighing about 6 ounces before broiling
2 brown-rice wafers *** with regular or low-calorie margarine
½ Broiled Grapefruit **
Decaffeinated coffee—fat-free or whole milk
Artificial sweetener

---

4 ounces sugar-free tomato juice
1 fried egg—nonstick pan only
2 ounces (before cooking) Bacon or Kosher Fry
Beef **
2 slices toasted soy-oat bread ***
Diet or regular margarine
Decaffeinated coffee—fat-free or whole milk
Artificial sweetener

---

1 apple baked with artificial sweetener, 1 tbs.
cherry soda (low-calorie)
6 ounces (before cooking) shell steak
1 rice wafer *** with cottage cheese
Decaffeinated coffee—hot milk
Artificial sweetener

½ cup fresh strawberries
½ cup Kellogg's Special K protein cereal
2 tbs. non-dairy milk or 3 ounces fat-free or whole
milk
Decaffeinated coffee—hot milk
Artificial sweetener

---

3 ounces orange juice
1 veal cutlet (3 ounces before cooking)
1 fried egg—nonstick pan only
1 slice soy-oat bread ***
Decaffeinated coffee—fat-free or whole milk or
non-dairy coffee creamer
Artificial sweetener

** See Recipe Index
*** Buy in Health Food Store

4 ounces fresh orange juice
2 shirred eggs and bacon
1 Gluten Soybean Muffin ** with regular or low-calorie margarine
Decaffeinated coffee—fat-free or whole milk
Artificial sweetener

---

4 ounces fresh or unsweetened canned orange juice
2 kosher frankfurters boiled or broiled—sugar-free mustard
1 slice sour rye bread—regular or low-calorie margarine
Decaffeinated coffee—fat-free or whole milk
Artificial sweetener

½ small grapefruit
Hamburger
2 brown-rice wafers ***
Regular or low-calorie margarine
Decaffeinated coffee—fat-free or whole milk
Artificial sweetener

Fruit cup of sliced oranges, grapefruit, grapes
1 scrambled egg and Canadian bacon
1-½ slices whole wheat bread with cottage cheese
Decaffeinated coffee or weak tea—fat-free or whole milk
Artificial sweetener

---

4 ounces unsweetened apple juice
1 scrambled egg with 2 ounces chicken livers
1 slice oatmeal bread with regular or low-calorie margarine
Decaffeinated coffee or weak tea—fat-free or whole milk
Artificial sweetener

** See Recipe Index
*** Buy in Health Store

4 ounces fresh or unsweetened canned orange
  juice
1 3-ounce slice cooked, cold pot roast
1 slice soy-oat bread ***
2 tbs. sugar-free peanut butter ***
Decaffeinated coffee—fat-free or whole milk
Artificial sweetener

---

4 ounces sugar-free tomato juice
5 ounces Filet of Sole Meunière **
2 rice wafers
1 ounce cottage cheese
Decaffeinated coffee—fat-free or whole milk
Artificial sweetener

---

1 tangerine
2 baby lamb chops
Fried Potatoes HG **
Decaffeinated coffee—fat-free or whole milk
Artificial sweetener

---

1 cup blueberries
3 ounces fat-free or whole milk
2 artichoke flour biscuits *** with 1 tbs. cottage
  cheese
Decaffeinated coffee—fat-free or whole milk
Artificial sweetener

½ banana—¼ cup raspberries
3 ounces plain, fat-free yogurt with artificial
  sweetener to taste
2 blueberry muffins—cottage cheese
Decaffeinated coffee—hot milk
Artificial sweetener

** See Recipe Index
*** Buy in Health Food Store

5163515

RUTLAGE J BRAZEE

07/84 VISA

#PCS 21 1165/RCKVLL MD
AMBULATORY CARE PHCY
8163172 219069
19860 98447 1122

THIS FORM TO BE USED WITH

MasterCard OR VISA®

SALES SLIP

991-7018

SALES SLIP

QTY.	CLASS	DESCRIPTION	PRICE	AMOUNT
		Tetra-Mycs		
		Ascreptin		
			SUB TOTAL	
			TAX	
			TOTAL	22.16

DATE 10/3/83

AUTHORIZATION   CLERK   REG./DEPT.

The issuer of the card identified on this item is authorized to pay the amount shown as TOTAL upon proper presentation. I promise to pay such TOTAL (together with any other charges due thereon) subject to and in accordance with the Agreement governing the use of such card.

CUSTOMER SIGNATURE X _____

AMBULATORY CARE

PHARMACY
424-1411

OCT 13 '83 J.N.

(ADJACENT TO SHADY GROVE ADVENTIST HOSPITAL)

9715 MEDICAL CENTER DR. ROCKVILLE, MD 20850

DATE 10-13-83	PHYSICIAN		
NAME			
ADDRESS			
	tolyt pads		8 10
	Ascription		17 07
			25 17
			-2 51
			22 66
		TAX	
RECEIVED BY		TOTAL	

3 *ounces sugar-free tomato juice*
Broiled veal chop
6 *canned asparagus*
1 *fresh sliced peach*
6 *fresh cherries*
Decaffeinated coffee—fat-free or whole milk or
non-dairy coffee creamer
Artificial sweetener

---

1 *cup stewed rhubarb with artificial sweetener to*
taste
3 *ounces fat-free plain yogurt*
1 *poached egg on 1 slice whole-wheat toast*
Decaffeinated coffee—fat-free or whole milk
Artificial sweetener

½ *cup blueberries*
2 *ounces fat-free or whole milk*
Artificial sweetener
2 *slices toasted soy-oat bread* ***
2 *tbs. natural peanut butter* ***
1 *tbs. low-calorie margarine*
Decaffeinated coffee—fat-free or whole milk
Artificial sweetener

---

1 *cup fresh or unsweetened canned blueberries*
Artificial sweetener to taste
4 *ounces plain yogurt*
Decaffeinated coffee—fat-free or whole milk
Artificial sweetener

---

3 *ounces fresh grapefruit juice*
5-*ounce shell steak (after cooking)*
½ *Broiled Grapefruit* **—*artificial sweetener*
Decaffeinated coffee—fat-free or whole milk
Artificial sweetener

** *See Recipe Index*
*** *Buy in Health Store*

3 ounces unsweetened prune juice ***
5 ounces baked or broiled ham steak
1 slice soy-oat bread ***, toasted or plain
1 tbs. cottage cheese
Decaffeinated coffee—fat-free or whole milk
Artificial sweetener

---

1 cup watermelon balls with 1 ounce plain yogurt
Mock French Toast **
Decaffeinated coffee—hot milk
Artificial sweetener

½ cup unsweetened applesauce
2 Poached Eggs à la Cheddar **
1 ounce Bacon or Kosher Fry Beef **
Brown-rice wafer ***, heated
Regular or low-calorie margarine, or butter
Decaffeinated coffee—fat-free or whole milk
Artificial sweetener

---

3 ounces unsweetened apple juice
1 poached egg
1 ounce Bacon or Kosher Fry Beef **
2 slices soy-oat bread ***
Regular or low-calorie margarine, or butter
Decaffeinated coffee—fat-free or whole milk
Artificial sweetener

---

2 halves dietetic peaches ***
1 egg-cheese omelet
1 slice soy-oat bread ***
Regular or low-calorie margarine, or butter
Decaffeinated coffee—fat-free or whole milk
Artificial sweetener

** See Recipe Index
*** Buy in Health Food Store

¼ papaya
3 ounces (before cooking) broiled halibut, cold or
   hot
1 cup chopped spinach
1 Strawberry Muffin **
Regular or low-calorie margarine, or butter
Decaffeinated coffee—fat-free or whole milk
Artificial sweetener

---

1 cup raspberries, blackberries, or blueberries
1 tsp. Vigorella ***
6 ounces plain fat-free yogurt
½ slice soy-oat bread ***
1 tbs. cottage cheese
Decaffeinated coffee—fat-free or whole milk
Artificial sweetener

---

2 ounces grapefruit juice, fresh or unsweetened
   canned juice
1 poached egg
2 Raspberry Muffins **
Regular or low-calorie margarine
Decaffeinated coffee—hot milk
Artificial sweetener

---

2 frankfurters boiled or broiled
Fried turnips
Chopped spinach
Bing Bang Jello **
Decaffeinated coffee—regular or fat-free milk
Artificial sweetener

½ cup raspberries with two ounces milk, and
   artificial sweetener
4-ounce shell steak (after cooking)
1 Blueberry Muffin **
Low-calorie or regular margarine or butter
Decaffeinated coffee—black

** See Recipe Index
*** Buy in Health Food Store

1 sliced fresh peach or 2 halves dietetic canned
peaches, with 2 ounces milk and artificial sweetener, if desired
4 ounces cold broiled salmon or halibut
1 slice Gluten-Oat Bread ** with pat of low-
calorie or regular margarine or butter
Decaffeinated coffee—fat-free or whole milk, or
cream
Artificial sweetener

¾ cup blueberries, topped with a small ball cottage cheese and 4 ounces plain yogurt (artificially sweetened, if desired)
Iced decaffeinated coffee with fat-free or whole
milk, or cream
Artificial sweetener

½ cup unsweetened applesauce
2 Poached Eggs à la Cheddar **
1 ounce Bacon or Kosher Fry Beef
Brown-rice wafer ***, heated
Regular or low-calorie margarine, or butter
Decaffeinated coffee—fat-free or whole milk
Artificial sweetener

---

3 ounces unsweetened apple juice
1 poached egg
1 ounce Bacon or Kosher Fry Beef **
2 slices soy-oat bread ***
Regular or low-calorie margarine, or butter
Decaffeinated coffee—fat-free or whole milk
Artificial sweetener

---

2 halves dietetic peaches ***
1 egg-cheese omelet
1 slice soy-oat bread ***
Regular or low-calorie margarine, or butter
Decaffeinated coffee—fat-free or whole milk
Artificial sweetener

** See Recipe Index
*** Buy in Health Food Store

3 ounces unsweetened apple juice
1 poached egg
1 ounce Bacon or Kosher Fry Beef **
2 slices soy-oat and oatflour bread ***
Butter, diet or regular margarine
Decaffeinated coffee, hot milk, artificial sweetener

---

4 ounces fresh grapefruit juice
1 Zucchini Omelet **
Blueberry Muffin **
Diet margarine or butter
Decaffeinated coffee—milk or cream
Artificial sweetener to taste

** See Recipe Index
*** Buy in Health Food Store

Lunch Delight Menus

These are quickly and easily prepared and adaptable to the
different seasons.

*Avocado pears with cottage cheese and dill on bed
of romaine salad garnished with watercress,
celery hearts and carrot sticks. Our HG Salad
Dressing ***
Cranberry Muffins **
Bing Bang Jello **
Decaffeinated coffee—fat-free or whole milk
Artificial sweetener

---

*4 ounces of sugar-free apricot juice *** (arti-
ficial sweetener can be added, if desired)*
Filet of sole (lemon flounder)
Broccoli with Hollandaise Sauce **
Caribbean Custard **
Decaffeinated coffee—fat free or whole milk
Artificial sweetener

---

2 baby lamb chops
Artichoke Flour Shells HG Style **
Fruit salad
Plum Muffins **
Decaffeinated coffee—fat free or whole milk
Artificial sweetener

** See Recipe Index
*** Buy in Health Food Store

16

Sliced cold turkey
Baked tomato with chopped artichoke bottoms
Chopped spinach
Strawberry Whip **
Decaffeinated coffee—fat-free or whole milk and artificial sweetener if desired

---

½ avocado stuffed with cottage cheese and chives
Carob Mousse **
Decaffeinated coffee—fat-free or whole milk, artificial sweetener, if desired

---

Hot chicken consommé (½ cup for HG people)
Hamburger
Chopped spinach
Asparagus tips with slices of green and red pepper vinaigrette
Apples baked with artificial sweetener to taste
Decaffeinated coffee—fat-free or whole milk
Artificial sweetener

---

4 ounces sugar-free tomato juice
Water-packed salmon—individual can, approximately 3-¼ ounces
Asparagus tips vinaigrette
Plain muffins, peanut butter with chopped apples
Decaffeinated coffee—fat-free or whole milk
Artificial sweetener

Jellied Chicken Ring **
Watermelon Balls with crème de menthe
Decaffeinated coffee—fat-free or whole milk
Artificial sweetener

** See Recipe Index

Tuna Ring **
Spinach soufflé
*Mixed green salad with low-calorie Italian dress-
  ing* ***
Raspberry Muffins ** *with regular or low-calorie
  margarine, or butter*
Blueberry Mousse **
Decaffeinated coffee—fat-free or whole milk
Artificial sweetener

Jellied Consommé **
Salmon Salad HG Style **
Sliced plums, fresh or dietetic canned
*Weak iced tea with lemon, mint and artificial
  sweetener, or iced decaffeinated coffee with 2
  ounces fat-free or whole milk*
Artificial sweetener

---

4 ounces V-8 juice
*1 medium-sized scoop of cottage cheese with
  sprinkling of caraway seeds on bed of lettuce.
  ½ tomato cut in wedges. Plain yogurt as topping or our HG Salad Dressing* **
Tangerine
*Weak iced tea with lemon, mint, and artificial
  sweetener, or iced decaffeinated coffee with fat-
  free or whole milk*
Artificial sweetener

Jellied tomato soup **
*Broiled kosher frankfurters (barbecue them if
  you like) with mustard*
Braised celery
*Lettuce with shredded cabbage and roasted al-
  monds, cottonseed oil and vinegar or Good
  Seasons Italian Dressing*
Melon in season
Decaffeinated coffee—fat-free or whole milk
Artificial sweetener

** See Recipe Index
*** Buy in Health Food Store

4 ounces sugar-free tomato juice
Peanut butter and Bacon or Kosher Fry Beef **
    on toasted Gluten-Oat Bread **
Dill pickles
Blackberry Sponge **
Decaffeinated coffee—fat-free or whole milk
Artificial sweetener

Avocado pears stuffed with cottage cheese and
    chives
Decaffeinated Coffee Jello **
Decaffeinated coffee—fat-free or whole milk
Artificial sweetener

Cold sliced roast beef
String beans with roasted almonds
Key Lime Chiffon Jello in individual molds **
Iced tea with lemon, mint and artificial sweetener

---

3 ounces unsweetened apple juice
Cottage cheese and fruit salad **
Raspberry-Cottage Cheese Topping **
Iced tea with lemon, mint and artificial sweetener

Jellied Tomato Soup **
Salmon Ring **
Cauliflower with hollandaise or browned mar-
    garine sauce
Stuffed pears **
Decaffeinated coffee—fat-free or whole milk
Artificial sweetener

½ orange
2 poached eggs on one slice toasted Gluten-Oat
    Bread ** with Hollandaise Sauce **
Strawberry Frou Frou **

** See Recipe Index

4 ounces sugar-free tomato juice
*Cold Veal Salad ** on bed of lettuce, garnished
with cucumbers, tomato wedges and sections of
hard-boiled eggs, and radish rosettes*
Purple Heart Jello ** Grand Marnier
*Iced tea (weak), artificial sweetener, mint and
lemon, or 8 ounces diet fruit soda*

Pepburgers **
Raw spinach salad with Our HG Salad Dressing **
*Strawberry Muffins ** with low-calorie or regular
margarine, or butter*
*Sliced fresh peaches — yogurt — Black Cherry
Sauce ***
*Weak iced tea with wedge of 1 lemon, mint, and
artificial sweetener*

---

3 ounces unsweetened apple juice
3¼-ounce can water-packed tuna
*1 medium-sized scoop of cottage cheese with
topping of plain yogurt*
Key Lime Chiffon Jello **
Decaffeinated coffee—fat-free or whole milk
Artificial sweetener

Sliced cold turkey
Baked tomato with chopped artichoke bottoms
Chopped spinach
Strawberry Whip **
Decaffeinated coffee—fat-free or whole milk
Artificial sweetener

Jellied Chicken Ring **
Watermelon balls with crème de menthe
Decaffeinated coffee demitasse

** See Recipe Index

Cornish Hen or Chicken and Frankfurter Salad **
  on lettuce garnished with radishes, hard-boiled
  egg and cherry tomatoes
Baked Peaches or Nectarines **
Iced tea with mint and lemon
Artificial sweetener

Apple, Sharp Cheese and Soybean Balls **
4-ounce veal chop, broiled
Chopped frozen creamed spinach
Chocolate Bavarian **
Weak iced or hot tea—artificial sweetener if de-
  sired, lemon wedges

Large bowl Plum Soup **
Tossed salad
4 ounces yogurt
Iced tea (very weak)
Artificial sweetener to taste

---

3 ounces sugar-free tomato juice
1 small can salmon
1 ball cottage cheese, size depends on appetite
4 ounces yogurt with artificial sweetener to taste,
  poured over
¼ cup blueberries
Iced decaffeinated coffee, cream, regular or fat-
  free milk

Tunafish salad on lettuce with Mayo 7
1 slice Cranberry Bread **
Strawberry Whip **
Iced decaffeinated coffee with cream, regular or
  fat-free milk

** See Recipe Index

Ladies and Gentlemen: Dinner Is Served

Whether it's going to be *à deux*, buffet, or a glorious sitdown with your best glassware, china and table appointments, these menus will have the right appeal.

Mushrooms sautéed with almonds
Veal chops and grapes
Spinach soufflé
String bean salad
Melon Balls Crème de Menthe **
Decaffeinated coffee—fat-free or whole milk
Artificial sweetener

Jellied Beef Bouillon **
Roast Beef and Mustard **
Yellow Squash Pancakes **
Spinach Salad with Our HG Salad Dressing **
Blackberry Supreme **
Decaffeinated coffee—fat-free or whole milk
Artificial sweetener

Jellied bouillon
Broilers with grapes
Chopped spinach
Baby lima beans
Beets vinaigrette
Watermelon
Decaffeinated demitasse

*** See Recipe Index*

*Roast Cornish hen, rice wafer and mushroom
    stuffing
Eggplant Soufflé **
Avocado and spinach salad. Good Seasons Italian
    dressing, or oil and vinegar
Blueberry Pudding **
Decaffeinated coffee—fat-free or whole milk
Artificial sweetener*

---

*Jellied Beef Bouillon **
Sparkling Pot Roast **
Yellow Squash Pancakes **
Spinach salad with scallion chips and bite-sized
    tomatoes
HG Apricot Soufflé **
Decaffeinated coffee—fat-free or whole milk
Artificial sweetener*

SPECIAL OCCASION DINNER

*Artichoke Bottoms Stuffed with Chopped Veal **
Barbecued Cornish Hen
Artichoke Flour Shells **
Fresh Bing Cherry and Port Wine Mold (instead
    of cranberry sauce) **
Spinach salad with grapefruit wedges and sliced
    avocado
Midnight Pudding **
Decaffeinated coffee—fat-free or whole milk
Artificial sweetener*

---

*Asparagus tips on toasted Gluten-Oat Bread **
Tuna Ring **
Mushroom Sauce **
Broccoli with Hollandaise Sauce ** or yogurt and
    mustard sauce
Lima beans
Fresh fruit cup
Decaffeinated demitasse*

** See Recipe Index

Papaya
Baked Filet of Sole with White Grapes **
½ cup tiny whole beets
Endive Fromage **
Baked apple with artificial sweetener
HG Apricot Soufflé **
Decaffeinated coffee—fat-free or whole milk
Artificial sweetener

Fresh or canned asparagus tips hollandaise
Baked Veal Chops **
Artichoke Flour Shells **
Brussels sprouts sprinkled with peanuts
Endive salad, Our HG Salad Dressing **
Baked grapefruit with artificial sweetener and 1 teaspoon dry red wine
Decaffeinated coffee—fat-free or whole milk
Artificial sweetener

Manhattan clam chowder
Broiled lobster tails, diet or regular margarine, safflower oil, or butter
½ cup peas
Raw broccoli, Mock Hollandaise Sauce **
1 cup tossed salad, Our HG Salad Dressing **
Bing Bang Jello **
Decaffeinated coffee—fat-free or whole milk
Artificial sweetener

Mushrooms sautéed with chicken livers
Broiled lamb chops
String beans amandine (make your own roasted almonds or use prepared frozen combination)
Spinach and avocado salad
Apple Brown Betty HG **
Decaffeinated coffee—fat-free or whole milk
Artificial sweetener

*** See Recipe Index*

Creamed asparagus soup
Soft-shell crabs broiled with minimum margarine,
    butter or safflower oil
*Cauliflower, Hollandaise Sauce ***
Stuffed pears
*Decaff inated Coffee Jello ***
Decaf einated coffee—fat-free or whole milk
Artificial sweetener

---

*Broiled Grapefruit ***
*Chicken Fricassee ** with meatballs*
*Artichoke Flour Spaghetti ***
Brussels sprouts
*Key Lime Chiffon Jello ***
*Zabaglione HG Style ***
Decaffeinated coffee—fat-free or whole milk
Artificial sweetener

Low-calorie borscht with sour cream or yogurt
*Sweet and Sour Pot Roast ***
Frozen baby lima beans
Hot artichoke hearts
*Key Lime Chiffon Jello ***
Decaffeinated coffee—fat-free or whole milk
Artificial sweetener

Artichoke Salad
*Fresh Salmon Chablis ***
*Baked Acorn Squash ***
*Apple Brown Betty HG ***
Decaffeinated coffee—fat-free or whole milk
Artificial sweetener

---

*Artichoke Bottoms and Chopped Veal ***
*Ham and Chicken in Wine ***
Wax beans
Grapefruit and orange fruit cup with kirsch
Decaffeinated demitasse

*** See Recipe Index*

Mushrooms sautéed with almonds
Shell steak
Zucchini Casserole **
Spinach and Avocado Salad
Crêpes Suzette HG Style **
Decaffeinated coffee—fat-free or whole milk
Artificial sweetener

---

*Tomato stuffed with cheddar cheese on bed of
    lettuce*
Broiled red snapper with white wine and grapes
Panned Eggplant **
Endive salad, Our HG Salad Dressing **
Peach Mumbo-Jumbo **
Decaffeinated demitasse

Shrimp cocktail, HG Seafood Sauce **
Broiled porgy or striped bass
Chopped beet tops
Cold broccoli, Mock Hollandaise Sauce **
*Stringbeans and onion pearls salad, Our HG Salad
    Dressing* **
Purple Heart Jello Grand Marnier **
Decaffeinated coffee—fat-free or whole milk
Artificial sweetener

Mushrooms sautéed with almonds
Roast capon with grapes
Chopped spinach
Artichoke hearts vinaigrette
Watermelon balls
*Decaffeinated demitasse, milk or non-dairy
    creamer*
Artificial sweetener

** See Recipe Index

Cantaloupe
Cold brook trout (canned) on bed of lettuce,
*   lemon wedge, yogurt and Dill Sauce ***
Horseradish sauce or Mayo 7 with mustard
For the very careful, plain yogurt with lemon juice
Decaffeinated coffee

Roast Cornish hen
*Stuffing on side: Artichoke Flour Shells ** with*
*   fresh mushrooms*

String beans with toasted nuts
Spinach salad with sliced avocado, safflower oil
*   and vinegar dressing with dash of pepper and*
*   garlic salt*
*Bing Bang Jello **, Mock Whipped Cream*
*   Sauce ***
Decaffeinated coffee—fat-free or whole milk
Artificial sweetener

¼ cantaloupe
Cold boiled salmon, lemon wedges, garni
*Mushroom Sauce **, plain yogurt or horseradish*
*   sauce*
Italian beans
Baked potato
Lettuce and tomato salad, Good Seasons Italian
*   Dressing*
*Cheesecake ***
Decaffeinated coffee—fat-free or whole milk
Artificial sweetener

---

*Baked Artichoke Bottoms and Chopped Veal ***
Half broilers baked with orange juice and grapes
*Panned Eggplant ***
*Waldorf Salad HG ***
*HG Apricot Soufflé ***
Decaffeinated demitasse

*** See Recipe Index*

*Baked filet of sole or halibut cocktail, HG Seafood
    Sauce ***
Chicken Fricassee **
*Spinach salad with 2 or 3 slices grapefruit per
    portion, and sliced raw mushrooms*
Baked Peaches **
Decaffeinated coffee—fat-free or whole milk
Artificial sweetener

Artichoke Hollandaise **
Brook trout amandine
Cauliflower, Rice Wafer Sauce **
Hearts of Palm Salad **
Purple Heart Jello Grand Marnier **
Decaffeinated coffee—fat-free or whole milk
Artificial sweetener

Beef bouillon with brown rice wafer croutons
Veal and Almonds **
Mashed yellow squash
Stuffed tomato salad
Midnight Pudding **
Decaffeinated demitasse

Halibut cocktail HG Seafood Sauce **
Veal Cutlets au Vin **
Spinach soufflé
Tossed salad, Our HG Salad Dressing **
Strawberry Mousse **
Decaffeinated coffee—fat-free or whole milk
Artificial sweetener

Jellied Bouillon **
Broilers with grapes
Chopped spinach
Zucchini Casserole **
Tossed salad, our HG Salad Dressing **
Watermelon
*Decaffeinated demitasse, fat-free or whole milk,
    or cream*
Artificial sweetener

** See Recipe Index

Fresh trout with lemon wedges and watercress
Stuffed Zucchini **
Spinach soufflé
Tossed Salad, Our HG Salad dressing **
Caribbean Custard **
Decaffeinated coffee—fat-free or whole milk, or
  cream
Artificial sweetener

½ artichoke vinaigrette
Double lamb chops
Mashed broccoli
Zucchini, tomato and onion casserole
Apricot Delight Cake **
Decaffeinated coffee, or weak tea, whole or fat-
  free milk
Artificial sweetener to taste

Charcoal-broiled veal chops
Eggplant Souffle **
Fresh string beans
Spinach salad with grapefruit wedges and slices
  avocado
Blueberry Supreme **
Decaffeinated coffee—fat-free milk or whole milk
  or cream
Artificial sweetener

Jellied Consommé **
Barbecued broilers (½ to a person) with our Bar-
  becue Sauce **
Broccoli, Hollandaise Sauce ** on side
Tossed salad with Our HG Salad Dressing **
Strawberry Mousse ** framed with ladyfingers
Decaffeinated coffee—fat-free milk, whole milk or
  cream
Artificial sweetener

** See Recipe Index

Saumon Poissonade au Charbon de Bois **
Red-cap charcoal-broiled eggplant **
*Spinach salad with sliced raw mushrooms, our
    HG Salad Dressing* **
Caribbean Custard **
*Iced decaffeinated coffee, fat-free milk, whole milk
    or cream*
Artificial sweetener

Asparagus tips on toasted Gluten-Soy Bread **
Tuna Ring ** *with Mushroom Sauce* **
Broccoli with Hollandaise **, *yogurt or mustard
    sauce*
Lima beans
Strawberry Whip **
Decaffeinated coffee—fat-free or whole milk
Artificial sweetener

Mock Vichyssoise **
Baked Veal Chops ** *with pears*
Cauliflower hollandaise
Eggplant Soufflé **
*Scallion, cucumber and lettuce salad, Good Sea-
    sons Italian Dressing with safflower oil and
    vinegar*
Watermelon balls
Decaffeinated demitasse

Whole artichoke vinaigrette
Filet of Sole with White Grapes **
String beans with onions
Tossed Salad ** *with walnuts, Good Seasons Ital-
    ian Dressing with safflower oil and vinegar*
Blackberry Sponge ** *with whipped non-dairy
    topping*
Decaffeinated coffee—fat-free or whole milk
Artificial sweetener

*** See Recipe Index*

Chilled flaked halibut, HG Seafood Sauce **
Cornish hen stuffed with Artichoke Shells **
Acorn Squash with Grapes **
Tossed salad
Apple Brown Betty HG **
*Decaffeinated coffee with milk or weak tea with
   milk*
Artificial sweetener

Artichoke Hollandaise **
Stuffed Chicken Breasts **
String beans and almonds
Salad
*Assorted melon balls with blackberries and other
   fruit in season, sprinkled with raspberry brandy*
Decaffeinated demitasse

Cold Orange and Green Melon Soup **
Broiled veal chop
Chopped spinach with riced, hard-boiled egg
Salad, Our HG Salad Dressing **
Decaffeinated Coffee Jello **
Decaffeinated demitasse

Cold Apricot Soup **
Breaded Veal Cutlets **
Stringbeans
Cauliflower, brown butter or margarine sauce
Yogurt
Decaffeinated demitasse

Mushroom Soup Purée **
Veal and Mushrooms **
*Canned or fresh asparagus with or without hol-
   landaise*
*Iceberg lettuce with artichoke bottoms, sliced scal-
   lions—oil and vinegar dressing*
*Fresh fruit topped with yogurt put through
   blender*
Decaffeinated demitasse

*** See Recipe Index*

Menus

Hard cheese with Arti Stix ***
Broiled scrod with butter, or margarine
Spinach soufflé
Broccoli with Hollandaise Sauce **
Mock Blueberry Whip **
Decaffeinated demitasse

** See Recipe Index
*** Buy in Health Food Store

Appetizers and Snacks

APPLE, SHARP CHEESE AND SOYBEAN BALLS

½ cup sharp Cheddar, grated
½ cup apple, peeled and grated
½ cup crushed soybeans

Mix apple and cheese together. Form into balls with teaspoon. Roll in crushed soybeans. Set in refrigerator to chill. Pierce with toothpicks and serve. Yield: 10–12 balls.

MINIATURE CHINESE EGG ROLLS

½ cup sifted gluten flour
½ tsp. salt
1 cup water
2 eggs, slightly beaten
2 tbs. chopped onion or scallion
2 tbs. chopped celery
1 parsnip
1 tbs. cottonseed oil

6 water chestnuts, minced
1 tbs. bean sprouts (optional)
2 chopped mushrooms
½ cup cooked veal, minced
½ cup cooked shrimp, minced
1 tsp. salt
2 tbs. dry English mustard

Mix flour, salt, water and eggs in bowl, reserving 1 tbs. of beaten egg for sealing rolls. Beat mixture until smooth. Pour about 1 tbs. batter into lightly greased, medium-hot 4-inch skillet. Tip pan to cover bottom with batter. Cook on one side only about 1 minute. Turn out on flat surface, uncooked side up. Continue until batter has been used. Combine onion, celery, carrot and mushrooms, cook 2 minutes in salad oil. Add remaining ingredients, mix thoroughly. Place 1 tsp. mixture on each pancake. Fold in sides, roll pancake, sealing ends with reserved beaten egg. Chill 1 hour. Fry in deep fat (360 degrees) until golden brown. Drain on paper towel. Serve with mustard thinned with hot water to consistency of cream. Makes 16 rolls.

DEVILED EGGS WITH MUSTARD

Cut cold hard-boiled eggs in half, remove yolks. Blend with Mayo 7, salt, pepper, and dried mustard. Spoon mixture back into halves. Cut halves into quarters. Serve cold, on bed of lettuce.

To Keep Yourself From Nibbling Try This Refreshing, Palatable Beverage in the Afternoon and/or Before Going to Bed

ENERGY MILKSHAKE

Mix 3 ozs. of 99% fat-free milk with 2 tsp. of nonfat dried milk and one tsp. of Pro-Slim protein powder. (Consult your doctor before you use this powder, as it contains a tiny bit of sucrose as well as cocoa and malt.) Put the mixture in your blender and add 4 or 5 more ozs. of the milk, or half milk and half water. Add ½ tsp. of vanilla and blend for 5 minutes. Make this milkshake even more nutritious by adding 1 egg and/or 1 tsp. brandy.

HAM-CHEESE BALLS

½ cup grated Swiss cheese
½ cup minced cooked ham
　or corned beef
½ tsp. sugar-free
　mustard ***

1 egg yolk
Salt and pepper to taste
Chopped parsley or chives

Mix all the ingredients together except parsley or chives. Shape into balls (use teaspoon). Roll lightly in parsley or chives. Pierce with toothpicks and chill for two hours.

What to Eat Between Meals Presented a Problem Until I Began Dreaming up All Sorts of Combinations

PEANUT BUTTER WITH CHOPPED APPLE

If you have not had toast for breakfast, this is a very good snack at 11 A.M. and an easy one. It is also a good filler for celery as

*** *Buy in Health Food Store*

an hors d'oeuvre. If you are not allowed to eat the standard brands, you can get peanut butter at the health store entirely without salt and sugar, or only with salt. Mix the following: 2 level tsp. of peanut butter, 1 heaping tsp. of grated apple with the peel, 2 ozs. of milk mixed with 2 ozs. of water. Spread on the toast or use as a filler for celery.

DEMI PEANUT BUTTER AND BACON SANDWICH

Peanut butter, bacon and lettuce filling
4 heaping tbs. sugar-free peanut butter ***
3 slices crisp lettuce
2 half slices soy-oat bread ***

Sauté 8 slices bacon or fry beef in nonstick pan. Set on paper towel to drain fat. Place between 2 half slices of soy-oat bread. On 2 half slices of soy and oat bread per person spread peanut butter, 2 slices bacon and lettuce. This half sandwich with 4 ounces sugar-free soda is a satisfying midnight (or earlier) snack.

PEANUT MEATBALLS

Make meatballs out of ground chuck or tenderloin steak, minced onions, salt, pepper and steak seasoning. Roll balls over chopped peanuts. Sauté in diet, regular margarine or butter. Serve with toothpicks.

PEANUT BUTTER NUT BALLS

Mix 1 heaping tsp. peanut butter with ⅛ tsp. grated apple. Separate and pat into 4 balls. Sprinkle with chopped pecans and refrigerate. Have 2 balls for a midmorning snack with 4 ozs. milk. Make a dozen and serve with beverages.

*** *Buy in Health Food Store*

PEANUT VEAL BALLS

1 lb. ground veal
1 cup sugar-free crunchy
   peanut butter ***
1 medium onion, minced
4 tbs. sugar-free chili
   sauce ***

1-½ tsp. salt
⅛ tsp. white pepper
1 egg, beaten
2 tbs. safflower oil
2 8-oz. cans tomato sauce

Mix the veal, peanut butter, minced onion, chili sauce, salt and pepper, and egg. Shape into tiny balls (use teaspoon to get uniform size). Brown on all sides in hot fat. Remove meat and pour off fat. Return meat to skillet and cover with tomato sauce. Cover skillet and *simmer* for 20 minutes. Use as hors d'oeuvre or as a lunch dish. Excellent to have on hand for in-between-meal snacks. Makes about 30 balls.

When You Are with Friends Who Are Ordering Delicious Ice Cream Sodas and Gooey Sundaes, You Really Do Feel out of Things. There Is Not Much You Can Do About it in a Restaurant, but when You Are Serving Sodas and Sundaes at Home You Can Make a Drink for Yourself That Everyone Will Mistake for a Soda. And It Tastes Delicious!

RASPBERRY SODA HG

6 ozs. sugar-free
   raspberry or black
   cherry soda. (Be sure
   that the soda has been
   refrigerated before you
   use it.)

6 ozs. plain yogurt
7 good-sized fresh
   strawberries
2 packages artificial
   sweetener
½ tsp. vanilla

Put the ingredients in your blender on Whip or Shake for a good 5 minutes. Then pour the whole in a tall glass. It will not only look beautiful, but taste delicious.

*** *Buy in Health Food Store*

SHRIMP TIDBITS

1 lb. shrimp, cooked and
   cleaned
1 scallion, chopped
1 tsp. salt
1 tbs. sherry
2 eggs, slightly beaten

½ cup gluten flour
2 tsp. baking powder
3 or 4 water chestnuts,
   finely chopped
Shortening for deep frying

Cut shrimp into tiny pieces. Mix with remaining ingredients, except shortening. Heat shortening to 360 degrees and drop mixture by teaspoonful into fat. Fry until crisp and golden brown (about 4 minutes). Drain on paper towel. Serve immediately. Yield: about 2 dozen.

APPLE AND CHEESE

Cut a small apple in large, thick slices. Top each slice with a wedge of cheddar, Gruyere, or individual caraway cheeses. The last two are in 1-oz. packages, a sufficient amount for an in-between snack with fruit. Take with 4 ounces of fat-free or whole milk and have a nutritious bedtime snack.

STUFFED CELERY

Mix 1 oz. plain yogurt with 1 oz. Swiss cheese and 1 tbs. shelled and chopped pistachio nuts. Stuff celery with mixture. Enjoy with 4 ozs. sugar-free juice.

OTHER QUICK SNACKS

2 kosher cocktail frankfurters with sugar-free mustard, and 4 ounces tomato juice

Stuffed Artichoke Bottoms ** and ½ bottle sugar-free black cherry soda

4 ounces milk blended with artificial sweetener and 3 fresh strawberries

** *See Recipe Index*

Midget burgers with sugar-free ketchup as a filling—4 ozs. tomato juice

A good-sized handful of nuts

½ brown rice wafer spread with tuna—4 ozs. fat-free milk

For a Late Evening Snack or a Summer Breakfast

YOGURT WITH FRUIT

Put ½ container plain yogurt in blender with 1 cup mashed raspberries, blackberries or blueberries, and artificial sweetener to taste. Blend on Chop and then on Frappe for at least 5 minutes. Pour into tall, thin glass.

BEEF BOUILLON SNACK

Another When-You-Are-Not-Hungry Suggestion: 6 ozs. Hot Beef Bouillon Topped with ½ Brown Rice Wafer Crumbled.

Breads, Muffins and Biscuits

This Section Is Ours Alone. After a Period of Trial and Much Error, We Came up with Much-Needed Recipes for Bread, Muffins and Biscuits. We Feel This Section Is a Great Contribution to the Low-Blood-Sugar Diet.

BLACKBERRY MUFFINS

1 cup gluten flour ***
1 cup oat flour ***
4 tsp. baking powder
4 egg yolks
2 tbs. melted shortening
1-⅓ cups orange juice, water, fat-free milk, or buttermilk

4 egg whites (beaten stiff)
1 cup blackberries
Salt or salt substitute
Artificial sweetener equal to ½ cup sugar

Mix egg yolks, liquid, salt and shortening. Sift flour, sweetener and baking powder together and add to egg yolk mixture. Fold in egg whites, add berries. Spoon into muffin tins and bake in 350-degree oven for 12 to 15 minutes. Makes 16 muffins.

BLUEBERRY BREAD-CAKE

Here is a delicious bit of bakery with which you can vary your diet. If you add sweetener to taste it's a cake. Topped with whipped cream you'll have your sweet tooth well filled. With just a bit of sweetener for flavoring, you have a bread you'll love. Substitute fresh raspberries or blackberries in season.

2 cups gluten flour ***
3 tsp. baking powder
3 eggs, beaten
2 tbs. shortening
1-½ cups buttermilk

1 tsp. salt
1 cup blueberries
Artificial sweetener equal to ½ cup sugar or to suit your taste

In a large bowl sift all the dry ingredients together. Beat the eggs, add the milk and shortening. Combine with the flour and mix well. Fold in the blueberries. Pour into a greased 9 x 5 x 3-inch loaf pan and bake in a 350-degree oven for 45 minutes to 1 hour. Makes 1 loaf.

*** *Buy in Health Food Store*

BLUEBERRY MUFFINS

1 cup gluten flour ***
1 cup oat flour ***
4 tsp. baking powder
4 egg yolks
2 tbs. melted shortening
1-⅓ cups fresh grapefruit
    juice

4 egg whites (beaten stiff)
1 cup blueberries
Artificial sweetener equal to
    ½ cup sugar
1 tsp. salt

Mix egg yolks, juice, salt or salt substitute and shortening. Sift flour, sweetener and baking powder together and add to egg yolk mixture. Fold in beaten egg whites, add berries. Spoon into muffin tins and bake in a 350-degree oven for 12 to 15 minutes. Makes 16 muffins.

CRANBERRY BREAD

2 cups soy flour ***
½ tsp. soda
½ tsp. salt

Artificial sweetener equal to
    1 cup sugar
2 tsps. baking powder

Sift together above ingredients. Add:

1 egg, well beaten
2 tbs. hot water
½ cup cranberries, chopped
    (fresh)
A few seedless grapes,
    chopped

2 tbs. melted shortening
½ cup nut meats
½ cup orange juice,
    unsweetened or fresh

Bake in 9 x 5 x 3-inch loaf pan 1 hour and 10 minutes in 325-degree oven. Cool. Wrap in wax paper and store for awhile in refrigerator before using. Makes 1 loaf.

CRANBERRY MUFFINS

1 cup gluten flour ***
1 tbs. melted diet or
    regular margarine
2 tsp. baking powder
2 egg yolks
⅔ cup fruit juice, water, milk
    or buttermilk

½ tsp. salt
2 egg whites (beaten
    stiff)
Artificial sweetener equal to
    ½ cup sugar
1-½ cups fresh
    cranberries

*** *Buy in Health Food Store*

Sprinkle cranberries with artificial sweetener. Mix egg yolks, margarine, liquid and salt or salt substitute. To this add flour and baking powder which have been sifted together. Into this mixture fold the beaten egg whites. Add berries. Pour into muffin tins and bake in a 350-degree oven from 12 to 15 minutes. Yields 6 large or 8 medium muffins.

MOCK FRENCH TOAST

4 slices True HG bread **
2 eggs
¼ cup fat-free milk
Artificial sweetener equal to
    1 tbs. sugar
Dash salt
Artificially sweetened maple
    syrup
2 tbs. butter or margarine
Cinnamon

Combine eggs, milk, salt, and sweetener. Beat with a wire whisk. Melt butter or margarine in skillet. Dip bread in egg mixture, coat both sides. Cook until nice and brown. Sprinkle with cinnamon and a little sugar substitute. Pour syrup over all. Serves 1.

GLUTEN-OAT BREAD

1 tbs. dry yeast
¾ tsp. salt
1-½ cups fruit juice
½ cup oat flour ***
3 cups gluten flour ***

Dissolve yeast and salt in fruit juice in large bowl, add gluten flour and then oat flour. Mix well into soft dough. Cover with clean cloth and let rise until almost double its size. It is preferable to leave it overnight. Punch dough down and let rise again for 30 minutes. Shape into loaf and place in 9 x 5 x 3-inch loaf pan. Bake in 350-degree oven for 1 hour. Makes 1 loaf.

GLUTEN AND SOY BISCUITS

1 cup gluten flour ***
1 cup soy flour ***
2-½ tsp. baking powder
1 tsp. salt
⅓ cup shortening
¾ cup milk or water

** See Recipe Index
*** Buy in Health Food Store

Sift dry ingredients together. Cut in shortening or use liquid shortening. Add the milk or water and mix into a soft dough. Turn onto a lightly floured board and knead. Roll ½-inch thick and cut with a 2-inch cutter. Bake in 350-degree oven for 12 to 15 minutes. Serves 6.

GLUTEN AND SOY BREAD

1 tbs. dry yeast
Artificial sweetener equal to
    2 tsp. sugar
½ cup warm water
1 cup milk, buttermilk or
    water, warmed

1-½ tsp. salt
1 tsp. melted shortening
1-½ cups gluten flour ***
1-½ cups soy flour ***
1 tsp. diet margarine,
    melted

Combine the yeast, sweetener and water. Let it stand 5 minutes to activate yeast. Add the milk, salt, shortening and flour. Mix to a soft dough. Turn onto a lightly floured board and knead 20 times. Place in a warm place and cover. Let dough rise until double its size. Knead again and place in 9 x 5 x 3-inch loaf pan. Grease top with margarine. Cover and let rise for 1 hour. Bake in 350-degree oven for 1 hour. Makes 1 loaf.

GLUTEN SOYBEAN MUFFINS

⅓ cup soybean flour,
    sifted ***
⅔ cup gluten flour,
    sifted ***
¼ tsp. liquid artificial
    sweetener

2 tsp. baking powder
¼ tsp. salt
1 egg, beaten
2 tbs. corn oil
½ cup water

Sift dry ingredients together into a bowl. Mix beaten egg, corn oil, liquid sweetener and water together. Pour liquid into dry ingredients. Stir until dry ingredients are just moistened. Spoon quickly into greased muffin tin. Bake at 400 degrees for 12–15 minutes or until golden brown. Makes 6 large muffins.

Printed with permission of Chicago Dietetic Supply, Inc.

*** *Buy in Health Food Store*

GLUTEN SOYBEAN YEAST BREAD

1 packet dry yeast
¼ tsp. sugar or artificial sweetener equal to ¼ tsp. sugar
½ cup warm water
Combine above and let stand for 3–4 minutes to activate yeast.

1 cup warm water	1-¼ cups soybean flour, sifted ***
1 beaten egg	
1-½ tsp. salt	3 cups gluten flour, sifted ***
1 tbs. corn oil	
3 drops liquid artificial sweetener	1 tsp. diet margarine, melted

Combine all ingredients in the order listed. Reserve ½ cup gluten flour for flouring board while kneading. Knead bread well. (It will be slightly tacky.) Put in a warm place to rise until doubled in bulk. Punch down and knead again. Form into loaf and place in greased 9 × 5 × 3-inch loaf pan. Grease top of loaf with melted margarine. Cover with wax paper until double in bulk. Bake at 350 degrees for one hour. Remove from pan and place on wire rack to cool. Store in plastic bag. Makes 1 loaf.

Printed with permission of Chicago Dietetic Supply, Inc.

PEANUT BUTTER BISCUITS

1 cup oat flour, sifted ***	2 tbs. artificially sweetened maple syrup ***
¼ tsp. sea salt ***	
Artificial sweetener equal to 1-½ tbs. sugar	
1 beaten egg	6 tbs. cold water
3 heaping tbs. sugar-free peanut butter ***	2-½ tsp. baking powder

Combine dry ingredients and blend in peanut butter. Add cold water and beaten egg. Stir to make soft dough. It will be sticky. Shape into small biscuits and place on greased cookie pan. Bake in preheated oven, at 350 degrees, 15–20 minutes. Yield: 9 biscuits.

Note: *For peanut butter I recommend Elam brand.*

*** *Buy in Health Food Store*

PLUM MUFFINS

1 cup gluten flour ***
1 cup fresh plums coarsely
    chopped *
Artificial sweetener equal to
    ¼ cup sugar

2 tsp. baking powder
1 tbs. safflower oil
1 cup buttermilk
2 egg yolks
2 egg whites (stiffly beaten)

In a large bowl, mix the egg yolks, milk and safflower oil. Add the flour and baking powder which have been sifted together. Sprinkle sweetener on the plums and add to flour mixture. Fold in stiffly beaten egg whites. Pour into well-oiled muffin tins. Bake for 15 minutes in 350-degree oven. Yield: 6 large muffins or 8 smaller ones.

RASPBERRY MUFFINS

1 cup gluten flour ***
2 tsp. baking powder
2 egg yolks
1 tbs. melted shortening
⅔ cup fat-free milk,
    buttermilk or water

½ tsp. salt
2 egg whites (beaten
    stiff)
1-½ cups raspberries
Artificial sweetener equal to
    ½ cup sugar

Mix egg yolks, shortening, fruit juice and salt or salt substitute. To this add flour and baking powder which have been sifted together. Into this mixture fold the beaten egg whites. Add berries which have been sweetened with artificial sweetener. Spoon into muffin tins and bake in 350-degree oven from 12 to 15 minutes. Makes 8 muffins.

SOY BREAD LOAF

1 cup soy flour ***
1 tsp. salt
2 tsp. baking powder

1 tsp. shortening—diet or
    regular margarine
⅔ cup water
4 eggs separated

Combine all ingredients except egg whites. Beat egg whites and fold in last. Bake in a 9 × 5 × 3-inch loaf pan for 30 to 40 minutes in moderate (350-degree) oven. Makes 1 loaf.

* *You can substitute apricots or prunes for the plums.*
*** *Buy in Health Food Store*

STRAWBERRY MUFFINS

1 cup gluten flour ***
1 cup oat flour ***
4 tsp. baking powder
4 egg yolks
2 tbs. melted shortening
1-⅓ cups unsweetened
    papaya juice *** or
    buttermilk

4 egg whites (beaten
    stiff)
1 box strawberries
⅛ tsp. salt
Artificial sweetener equal to
    ½ cup sugar

Sweeten papaya juice or buttermilk with artificial sweetener. Then mix egg yolks, salt and shortening with liquid. Sift flour and baking powder together and add to egg yolk mixture. Fold in beaten egg whites, add berries. Spoon into muffin tins and bake in 350-degee oven for 12 to 15 minutes. Makes 16 muffins.

With Gluten and Soy and Flavoring We Produced

TRUE HG BREAD

3 cups gluten flour ***
½ cup soy flour ***
¾ tsp. salt
1 tbs. dry yeast

1-½ cups orange juice
    (room temperature)
2 pkgs. powdered sugar
    substitute

Dissolve yeast, sweetener, and salt in orange juice in large bowl. Sift soy flour and gluten flour together. Add to yeast. Mix well into soft dough. Cover with clean towel and let rise until it doubles its bulk. Punch down, cover as before and let rise 45 minutes more. Turn onto a lightly floured board, shape into loaf. Place in 9 × 5 × 3-inch loaf pan. Bake in 350-degree oven for 1 hour. Makes 1 loaf.

Suggestion: slice bread very thin even when toasting.

*** *Buy in Health Food Store*

Soups

POTAGE ASPERGES
(*Asparagus Soup*)

2 15-oz. cans asparagus
¼ tsp. thyme
¼ tsp. dill

Fresh chopped parsley for garnish

Place asparagus and liquid from cans in blender, add thyme and dill and blend for two minutes. Set in saucepan and heat to boiling point. Pour into soup cups and sprinkle with chopped parsley. Serves 4–6.

POTAGE ASPERGES À LA CRÈME

Drop dabs of heavy unsweetened whipped cream on each serving.

JELLIED BEEF BOUILLON

1 can beef bouillon
1 can water
1 envelope unflavored gelatin

1 tsp. freshly chopped parsley
2 tbs. dry sherry

Heat the bouillon and water to boiling point. Soften gelatin in 2 tbs. of cold water and add to the bouillon. Add sherry and then pour into soup cups and chill. Sprinkle with chopped parsley. Serves 4.

SOUP WITH BEEF AND VEGETABLES

2-½ lbs. beef (brisket, top round or bottom round)
Soup greens cut up julienne style:
    2 carrots
    ½ celery root
    ½ parsley root

2-½ qts. water
2 tbs. salt or salt substitute
1 lb. cabbage, cut up
1 white onion, sliced
1 cup stringbeans, cut up
Chopped watercress for garnish
1 cup starch-free shells ***

*** *Buy in Health Food Store*

Cut meat into slices 2 inches thick. Place with soup greens in hot salted water. Cover tightly. Boil on medium flame for 1-½ hours. Add cabbage, onion and stringbeans and boil 1 hour longer. Skim fat off soup. Add shells and continue cooking until shells are tender. Cube meat and place in individual soup dishes. Add soup and sprinkle with chopped watercress. Serves 4–6.

CAULIFLOWERSSOISE

6 leeks, thinly sliced
3 cups cauliflower, cubed
2 cans chicken broth
2 cups skimmed milk
2 tbs. chives, chopped

½ cup light cream or whole milk
1 tsp. salt
Pepper to taste

Combine leeks, using pulp and thick part of green stalk, cauliflower and chicken broth. Cook ½ hour or until vegetables are tender. Press pulp and liquid through fine sieve or use electric blender. Add milk or cream, salt and pepper to the purée and bring to boil. Chill thoroughly. Serve very cold, garnished with chives. Serves 8.

COLD CUCUMBER SOUP

¼ cup onion, sliced
2 cups cucumbers, diced, unpeeled
2 sprigs watercress
1 11-oz. can chicken consommé
⅛ tsp. pepper
¼ tsp. sugar-free mustard

2 tbs. quick-cooking artichoke flour shells ***, chopped
1 cup cold water
1 cup sour cream or sour cream substitute
Paprika

Place all ingredients except water in saucepan, bring to boil, cook about 15 minutes. Put through sieve or use blender. Add water and sour cream or sour cream substitute. Chill. Sprinkle with paprika. Makes 4 cups.

*** *Buy in Health Food Store*

JELLIED CONSOMMÉ

1 8-oz. can of chicken
   consommé
1 8-oz. can of water
1 envelope unflavored
   gelatin

1 tsp. freshly chopped chives
   or dill
2 tbs. dry white wine

Heat the consommé and water to boiling point in a saucepan. Soften gelatin in 2 tbs. of cold water and add to the consommé. Add wine. Pour mixture into soup cups and chill. Sprinkle with chopped chives or dill. Serves 2–4.

CUCUMBER SOUP

2 cups chicken stock
½ cup cucumber, peeled,
   seeded and diced
½ cup white chicken meat

½ cup whole milk
½ cup tiny canned shrimp
1 tsp. chervil
Salt and pepper to taste

Bring the chicken stock and cucumber to a boil. Simmer for 10 minutes. Place chicken meat and milk in blender. Blend until a thick liquid is obtained. Add to the cucumber mixture; add the shrimp, salt and pepper and heat. Do not boil. Pour into soup cups. Sprinkle with chervil. Serves 4.

MUSHROOM SOUP PURÉE

½ lb. mushrooms, sliced
4 cups water
4 tbs. powdered chicken-
   flavored broth

Dash white pepper
1 tsp. salt
½ tsp. chopped parsley
½ cup evaporated milk

Cook mushrooms in water until tender, about 10 minutes. Add seasonings. Place in blender and purée for 3 minutes. Return to the pot and add milk. Heat and pour into soup cups. Sprinkle with parsley. Serves 6–8.

QUICK SPINACH SOUP

1 10-oz. pkg. chopped frozen
    spinach, cooked
    according to package
    directions, drained
1 cup whole milk

½ tsp. salt
½ tsp. Italian seasoning
Yolk of 1 egg, hard-boiled
    and grated

Place spinach in blender, add the milk and seasonings. Purée for 2 or 3 minutes. Heat to boiling point. Serve in warmed soup cups and sprinkle with grated egg yolk. Serves 4.

SPINACH OR WATERCRESS SOUP

1 10-oz. pkg. fresh spinach
    or
2 bunches of watercress
½ tbs. margarine
⅛ tsp. nutmeg

Salt and pepper to taste
3 egg yolks
2 cups chicken broth or
    water
½ cup skimmed milk

Melt the margarine. Add the broth and spinach or watercress which has been chopped very fine. Cook until tender (approximately 10 minutes). Add the seasonings and mix well. Just before serving time combine the egg yolks and milk. Add to the soup. Heat well, but do not boil. Serve immediately. Serves 6–8.

SQUASH SOUP

4 medium-sized yellow
    squashes or zucchini
4 cups water
3 chicken bouillon cubes
2 ozs. sour cream or sour
    cream substitute, if
    desired

Dash garlic powder
Dash Tabasco
Salt and pepper to taste
Few dry roasted peanuts,
    minced

Scrub the zucchini. (Do not peel.) Cut into cubes and cook in water until tender. Place in blender or purée through a strainer. Add chicken bouillon cubes. Stir until completely dissolved. Add the garlic powder, Tabasco, salt and pepper. Serves 4. Note: If a thinner soup is desired, add a little more water. Taste and correct. This soup may be served hot or cold. Garnish with small dabs of sour cream, and peanuts.

JELLIED TOMATO SOUP

4 cups sugar-free tomato
   juice ***
⅛ tsp. Tabasco
2 envelopes unflavored
   gelatin

½ tsp. dill weed
½ cup cold water
Chopped parsley for garnish
Lemon slices for garnish

Combine tomato juice, Tabasco and dill weed. Heat to boiling point. Soften gelatin in cold water and add to tomato juice. Stir until dissolved. Pour into soup cups and chill for 4 hours. Garnish with slice of lemon and chopped parsley. Serves 4.

TOMATO SOUP À L'ORANGE

2 lbs. ripe red tomatoes
1 medium onion, sliced
1 bay leaf
6 peppercorns
1 strip of lemon peel
2-½ pints chicken stock
Salt to taste

2 tbs. diet margarine
3 tbs. gluten flour ***
Artificial sweetener to taste
1 cup skimmed milk
Peel of ¼ orange, very thinly
   peeled
1 tsp. chopped dill

Cut tomatoes into quarters. Put tomatoes and onion in heavy saucepan. Add bay leaf, peppercorns, lemon peel, orange peel and stock. Add salt, cover and bring to a boil. Simmer partly covered 30 minutes. Rub through a fine sieve. Melt margarine in same pot, blend in gluten flour, gradually add soup and chicken stock, stirring until thickened and smooth. Add artificial sweetener and simmer 5 minutes or longer if too thin. Add milk and serve garnished with chopped dill. Serves 2–4.

MOCK VICHYSSOISE

4 cups plain yogurt
½ cup chopped pecans or
   walnuts
2 cups diced zucchini

Salt and pepper to taste
1 tbs. caraway seeds
Chopped parsley

Place pecans, zucchini, salt, pepper and caraway seeds in blender for 1 minute. Combine with yogurt. Sprinkle with chopped parsley. Chill for 4 hours. Serves 4–6.

*** *Buy in Health Food Store*

Before preparing these delicious cold fruit soups, be sure to consult your doctor. Otherwise, we suggest that you make the soup your chief carbohydrate for the day and confine yourself to a high-protein diet.

APRICOT SOUP I

2 lbs. apricots
Juice of 1 lime
Juice of 1 lemon
Juice of ½ grapefruit
1 oz. heavy cream or yogurt
Artificial sweetener to taste

Peel and pit apricots. Put them in blender on Chop with all the other ingredients and blend for at least 4 minutes. Then put mixture on Frappé for about 8 minutes. Pour into soup cups and set in refrigerator to chill for about 2 hours. Serves 4–6. Garnish with whipped cream or yogurt and blueberries.

APRICOT SOUP II

2 lbs. apricots
Juice of 2 limes
½ cup sauterne or other
white wine
Dash salt and pepper
5 pkgs. of artificial
sweetener
Juice of ½ grapefruit
1 oz. heavy cream
2 tbs. artificially sweetened
grape syrup or grape
flavoring
Sugar-free whipped cream
or sour cream substitute
for garnish
Fresh raspberries and
blueberries for garnish
Artificial sweetener to taste

Peel apricots and remove pits. Add seasonings and juices and fresh cream. Put in blender on Frappé and blend for 10 minutes. Then pour into soup cups and chill. Serves 4. Garnish with sugar-free whipped cream or sour cream substitute, fresh raspberries or blueberries, sprinkled with artificial sweetener.

CHERRY SOUP

2 lbs. fresh cherries
Juice of 1 fresh grapefruit
1 cup dry red wine
Artificial sweetener equal to
¼ cup sugar
¼ cup lemon juice
1 tbs. unflavored gelatin
¼ cup sugar-free whipped
cream
8 white seedless grapes

Wash cherries. Remove pits. Place in blender with grapefruit juice, lemon juice, wine and sweetener. Blend on Purée until smooth. Soften gelatin in a cupful of the purée and return to the blender. Blend for 2 minutes longer. Pour into soup cups and chill. Top with whipped cream and white grapes. Serves 4.

ORANGE AND GREEN MELON SOUP

½ honeydew melon
Juice of 1 lemon
Juice of 1 lime
 3 pkgs. artificial sweetener
Juice of half a grapefruit
 4 oz. sauterne
Dash nutmeg

1 tsp. artificial or imitation
  black walnut flavoring
½ cup sugar-free whipped
  cream, sour cream or
  sour cream substitute
12 small cantaloupe balls
Fresh chopped mint

Cut melon in chunks. Remove seeds and skin. Place in blender. Add lemon and lime juice, grapefruit juice, sweetener, nutmeg, wine and flavoring. Blend on Purée until smooth. Pour into four individual soup cups. Chill. When ready to serve, garnish with melon balls, dabs of whipped cream, sour cream or sour cream substitute, and fresh chopped mint. Serves 4. You can reverse this and have cantaloupe soup with honeydew melon balls.

PINK MELON SOUP

½ honeydew melon
½ cantaloupe
 1 cup fresh raspberries
Juice of 1 lemon
Juice of 1 lime
3 or 4 pkgs. artificial
  sweetener
Juice of ½ grapefruit
 4 oz. sauterne

Dash nutmeg
 1 tsp. artificially sweetened
  grape syrup
½ cup sugar-free whipped
  cream, sour cream or
  sour cream substitute
12 small watermelon balls
  or 12 bing cherries
Fresh chopped mint

Cut melons. Remove seeds and skin. Place in blender. Add raspberries, juices, wine, nutmeg, artificial sweetener and grape syrup. Blend on Chop and on Frappé for 7–10 minutes. Pour into individual soup cups and chill. Serves 4. When ready to serve, dab with whipped cream, sour cream or sour cream substitute, watermelon balls or cherries, and chopped mint. You can reverse this and have all honeydew or cantaloupe topped with balls of the other melon.

NECTARINE SOUP

2 lbs. nectarines
¼ cup sweet cream
Juice of 1 lemon
Juice of ½ grapefruit
1 tbs. imitation coconut
flavor
Blueberries for garnish

Sugar-free whipped cream
for garnish
¼ cup raspberries
5 pkgs. artificial sweetener
or less, according to
taste
½ cup dry red wine

Peel and pit nectarines. Place in blender on Chop for 4 minutes. Add juices, raspberries, sweet cream, wine, coconut flavor and artificial sweetener. Blend on Frappé for 7 to 10 minutes. Pour into soup cups and chill. When ready to serve, garnish with raspberries and dabs of whipped cream. Serves 4.

PLUM SOUP

2 lbs. plums
Juice of 1 lime
Juice of ½ grapefruit
1 cup dry red wine
1 pan boiling water
1 pan ice water

1 tbs. artificial caramel
flavoring
¼ cup sour cream or sour
cream substitute
¼ cup blueberries
4 pkgs. of artificial sugar

Place the plums in a pan of boiling water. Then plunge into ice water. Remove skins and pits. Place in blender, add lime juice, artificial sweetener, grapefruit juice, artificial caramel flavoring and wine. Blend until smooth. Pour into soup cups, chill. Garnish with berries and sour cream. Serves 4.

Salads

APRICOT SURPRISE

8 raw apricots
Lemon juice or Our HG
   Salad Dressing **
3 ozs. cream cheese
½ cup chopped walnuts

½ cup diced celery
Mayo 7 to taste
¼ cup chopped pistachio
   nuts
4 ozs. diet fruit juice

Peel apricots, cut in half, remove pits. Sprinkle with lemon juice or Our HG Salad Dressing. Fill the hollows with a mixture of cream cheese, chopped walnuts and diced celery. Press the halves together, arrange on lettuce leaves. Serve with Mayo 7 sweetened with diet fruit juice and sprinkled with chopped pistachio nuts. Serves 4.

ARTICHOKE SALAD

1 large head iceberg lettuce
1 can artichoke hearts
1 medium-sized cucumber
2 ripe tomatoes

1 cup Our HG Salad
   Dressing **
Salt and pepper to taste

In a large salad bowl break the lettuce into bite-sized pieces. Peel and slice cucumber, cut the tomatoes into eighths. Drain the artichokes and cut into halves. Pour over dressing, add salt and pepper to taste. Toss well. Serves 8–10.

CHICKEN SALAD

1 cup cooked chicken
½ cup diced celery
½ cup diced pineapple
Our HG Salad Dressing **

Lettuce leaves
Mayo 7
1 tsp. capers

Mix the chicken, celery, pineapple, moisten with dressing and let stand in refrigerator for 1 hour. Arrange in mounds on let-

** *See Recipe Index*

tuce leaves, top with a dab of Mayo 7 and sprinkle with capers. Serves 4.

CORNISH HEN OR CHICKEN AND FRANKFURTER SALAD

3 cups diced cooked poultry
2 frankfurters, boiled and
    sliced
3 scallions, chopped,
    including greens
2 tbs. chopped celery
1 tsp. salt
⅛ tsp. pepper.
Pinch herb blend for
    salads*

Generous sprinkling Sovex
    Bakon-Yeast Powder
Enough Mayo 7 to hold
    mixture together
1 hard-boiled egg, cut in
    wedges
4 radish rosettes
1 medium-sized tomato, cut
    in wedges

Combine diced poultry, frankfurters, scallions and celery. Add salt, pepper, herb blend, Bakon-Yeast Powder and toss. Then add Mayo 7 and mix. Set mixture on platter with lettuce. Garnish with hard-boiled egg wedges, radish rosettes and tomatoes. Pour Our HG Salad Dressing ** over lettuce if desired. Serves 4–6.

JELLIED CHICKEN RING

4 envelopes unflavored
    gelatin
2 cans clear chicken soup
1 cup Mayo 7
1 cup celery, finely chopped
½ cup red pepper
1 cup green pepper, finely
    chopped

1 cup sliced avocado,
    diced
½ cup chopped pecans
1-½ cups cooked chicken,
    diced
4 tbs. lemon juice
Diet margarine or safflower
    oil

Soften gelatin in cold water. Heat chicken soup and dissolve gelatin in it. Cool. When it is slightly thickened fold in other ingredients. Pour into ring mold well greased with margarine or safflower oil. Chill until firm. Serves 4–6.

* We recommend Wagner's
** See Recipe Index

COTTAGE CHEESE CARAWAY SALAD

8 ozs. low-calorie cottage
  cheese sprinkled with
  caraway seeds
2 tbs. plain yogurt—optional
3 avocados

6 crisp lettuce leaves
¾ cup Mayo 7
¾ cup diced cucumbers
1 cup (3 large stalks) diced
  celery

Combine cottage cheese, celery, cucumbers and Mayo 7. Mix lightly. Pare avocados, cut in half lengthwise and remove pits and dark patches. Fill with cottage cheese mix and serve on lettuce leaves.* Top each portion with yogurt, if desired. Serves 4–6.

COTTAGE CHEESE AND FRUIT SALAD

8 ozs. low-calorie cottage
  cheese
Several lettuce leaves

2 cups blueberries
Watermelon
2 ozs. orange juice

Spread lettuce leaves on plate. With small ice cream scoop, make 6 watermelon balls. Cut in half. Set flat portion in center of lettuce. With large ice cream scoop, make 6 balls of cottage cheese. Set each one on melon. Place ½ pear on either side of cottage cheese. Fill generously with blueberries. Cut remaining pear halves into quarters. Serves 4–6.

TANGY CRANBERRY MOLD

2 cups fresh cranberries
1 orange, peeled
½ cup walnuts
⅛-oz. can dietetic crushed
    pineapple
2 ozs. orange juice

2 tbs. artificially sweetened
  raspberry syrup
2 envelopes unflavored
  gelatin
2 tbs. cold water

Put through a meat grinder the cranberries, orange and walnuts, add the drained pineapple. Add the orange juice and raspberry syrup to the pineapple juice, enough to make 1 cup liquid. Heat this liquid. Soften gelatin in cold water and add to the hot

* Chives or 1 cup chopped salted peanuts may be substituted for the celery and cucumber.

liquid. Stir until dissolved. Combine all the ingredients. Pour into mold and chill. Serve with chicken, turkey or veal. Serves 8–10.

FRUIT SALAD PLATE

Place small lettuce leaves on large platter to form cups. Fill with fruit as follows:

Segments of orange and grapefruit
Mixed melon balls
Whole strawberries
Pineapple chunks sprinkled with chopped mint
Diet cream cheese and low-calorie cottage cheese balls, sprinkled with paprika
Pitted cherries stuffed with cut meats
Peanut butter balls rolled in chopped nuts

Make enough lettuce cups so that each person will have one of each fruit.

GREEN BEAN PARMESAN SALAD

2 lbs. green beans cut in 2-inch pieces
1 small onion, minced
½ cup safflower oil
¼ cup wine vinegar
1 tsp. salt
¼ tsp. pepper
½ cup grated Parmesan cheese

Cook beans in boiling salted water until tender. Drain and cool. Combine the remaining ingredients and pour over beans. Toss and serve. Serves 10.

HALIBUT SALAD

1 cup cooked flaked halibut
1 cup diced celery
Our HG Salad Dressing **
Lettuce leaves
Mayo 7
2 tbs. shredded green pepper
2 tbs. pimiento

Mix the halibut and celery, moisten with dressing and let stand in refrigerator for 1 hour. Arrange in mounds on cup-shaped lettuce leaves, garnish with green pepper and pimiento. Top with a dab of Mayo 7. Serves 3–4.

** *See Recipe Index*

LEFTOVER SALAD

2 cups cooked Cornish hen or
    turkey, cut up into large
    chunks
1 cup celery cut up in ¼-inch
    slices
1 tbs. lemon juice
Salt to taste
Dash seasoned pepper

Drained cut-up unsweetened
    pineapple (medium-
    sized can)
½ cup almonds with or
    without salt
Mayo 7 to moisten (about
    ½ cup)

Mix all ingredients with Mayo 7. Place on lettuce leaves. Garnish with deviled egg cut in quarters and cucumber wedges. Serves 6.

LIME MOLD

2 envelopes unflavored
    gelatin
½ cup lime juice
2 cups water
1 cup clear chicken soup
⅛ tsp. artificial sweetener

1 drop green food coloring
1 cup hearts of palm, sliced
½ cup cooked string beans
2 strips red pimiento, sliced
6 tiny whole beets for color
Radish rosettes, for garnish

Soften gelatin in 2 tbs. water. Heat chicken soup and remainder of water. Add softened gelatin and stir until dissolved. Add lime juice, sweetener and food coloring while stirring. Pour mixture into a 1-½-quart ring mold. Carefully drop in the vegetables, separating the colors to make mold look attractive. Place mold in refrigerator for 6 hours. Unmold to platter. Fill hole with watercress and garnish around mold with sprigs of parsley and radish rosettes. Serves 6–8.

LUNCHEON ASPIC SALAD

2 cups grapefruit sections
    (if canned, sugar-free)
3 spears white asparagus
    (canned)
½ lb. cooked shrimp (small)
2 tbs. unflavored gelatin
2 chicken bouillon cubes

3 cups liquid (juice from
    grapefruit, ¼ cup
    lemon juice, and enough
    water to make 3 cups of
    liquid)
¼ cup lemon juice
½ tsp. salt
2 tbs. capers

Peel and section the grapefruit or use canned grapefruit. Cut the asparagus into 1-inch pieces. Soften gelatin in a little of the juice mixture. Heat the remaining liquid to boiling point. Add bouillon cubes. Stir in softened gelatin. Mix until dissolved. Add salt. Place in refrigerator until it starts to gel. Sprinkle bottom of a 2-quart salad mold with capers. Spoon some of the gelatin mixture over the capers. Make layers of grapefruit, asparagus and shrimp until all the ingredients are used up. Chill, unmold, and serve. Serves 4–6.

MUSHROOM-SPINACH SALAD

10 oz. fresh spinach, stems removed

1 bunch scallions, cut up into tiny pieces
6 mushrooms, raw

Wash and shake spinach in large plastic bag; then dry with paper towel. Transfer spinach into smaller plastic bag and store in refrigerator. Wash and slice mushrooms in circular form after removing stems. Pour dressing that follows into bag with spinach mixture and shake to coat leaves. Just before serving remove spinach with dressing from bag and spread leaves on half-moon or ordinary glass plates. Spread mushrooms over leaves; scatter scallions over top and serve. Serves 6.

Dressing

½ onion
1 tsp. Dijon or other sugar-free mustard
½ tsp. sea salt

2 tbs. safflower oil
3 tbs. cider vinegar
Small amount lemon juice
Pinch dry mustard

Grate onion. Add seasonings, vinegar, lemon juice, Dijon and dry mustard. Stir and pour into pint bottle. Shake vigorously.

ORANGE-BEAN MOLD

1 pkg. unflavored gelatin
1 cup boiling water
1 cup fresh orange juice, strained
½ cup Mayo 7
Dash salt

Dash pepper
1-½ to 2-½ cups diced celery
½ cup sliced radishes
½ cup string beans (raw)— nice and crisp
1 bunch watercress

Melt gelatin in tablespoon cold water. Add 1 cup boiling water and orange juice in bowl. Blend all ingredients except celery, beans and radishes with a beater. Place in mold and refrigerate for 20 minutes until mixture starts to thicken. Pour in celery, beans and radishes artistically, so that they are spread around mold. Chill until set. Remove from mold onto round plate. Fill center with watercress and serve. Serves 6.

HEARTS OF PALM SALAD

3 14-oz. cans hearts of palm
2 avocados
2 heads iceberg lettuce

1 cup Our HG Salad
   Dressing **
Salt and pepper as desired

Break the lettuce into bite-sized pieces. Peel and dice the avocados. Cut the hearts of palm into ¼-inch pieces. Place in a large salad bowl. Pour over the dressing, add salt and pepper as desired. Toss gently. Serves 8–10.

STUFFED PEARS

8 diet canned pear halves
½ cup minced celery
2 tbs. Mayo 7

½ cup pistachio nuts
3-4 lettuce leaves

Place 8 diet canned pear halves on lettuce leaves. Stuff centers of fruit with minced celery mixed with Mayo 7. Top with chopped pistachio nuts. Serves 4.

RED COLD SALAD

1 envelope unflavored
   gelatin
16 ozs. low-calorie borscht
2 tbs. vinegar
2 tsp. grated onion
¼ tsp. salt
¼ tsp. dry mustard

Artificial sweetener equal to
   2 tbs. sugar
1 tbs. horseradish
1 cup canned tiny whole
   beets
½ cup green pepper, chopped
½ cup celery, chopped

Mix gelatin with cold water to soften. Then mix with 1 cup boiling water. Add borscht, vinegar, onion, salt, mustard, sweetener and horseradish. Cool. As mixture thickens add beets, green pepper and celery. Pour into greased mold and chill until firm. Serves 4–6.

** *See Recipe Index*

SALMON SALAD HG STYLE

1 salmon steak or 1 8-oz.
  can of salmon
2 tbs. finely chopped
  celery
1 tbs. finely chopped onion

¼ tsp. salt
Dash white pepper
2 tbs. Mayo 7
1 hard cooked egg, sliced
Lettuce leaves

Flake the salmon or put through a food grinder, using the coarse blade. Mix in the celery, onion, salt, pepper and Mayo 7. Shape into balls. Place on lettuce leaves and garnish with egg slices. Serves 4–6.

TOSSED SALAD

½ head small iceberg lettuce
½ head chicory
½ cup diced celery
¼ cup sliced scallions
1 tsp. chives
1 tsp. sea salt ***

Dash white pepper and garlic
  salt
1 large or 2 small yellow
  squashes
Dash herb blend for salads *
Our HG Salad Dressing **

Cut up iceberg lettuce and chicory into salad bowl. Add diced celery, sliced scallions, teaspoon chives, dash of herb blend for salads, sea salt and slices of yellow squash. Sprinkle salad with garlic salt and pepper and set in refrigerator. Immediately before serving, add HG dressing. Remember to shake bottle vigorously. Serves 4–6.

COLD VEAL SALAD

3-½ cups diced cold roast veal
½ cup chopped celery
1 cup scallions, sliced fine
1 tbs. chopped green
  pepper
1 heaping tbs. Mayo 7
½ iceberg lettuce
¼ Bibb lettuce
Our HG Salad Dressing **

½ tsp. salt
⅛ tsp. pepper
Dash garlic salt
Sprinkling chives
Dash herb blend for salad *
6 radish rosettes
½ bunch watercress
1 cucumber

* We recommend Wagner's
** See Recipe Index
*** Buy in Health Food Store

Mix veal, celery, scallions and green pepper in bowl. Add salt, pepper, garlic salt, herb blend for salad and sprinkling of chives. Put in Mayo 7 to hold salad together and mix well. On oval or oblong platter, spread iceberg lettuce, saving Bibb lettuce for each end. Peel and slice cucumber thin. Scatter slices at either end of platter. Make radish rosettes (or just slice radishes) and place among cucumbers. Set mix in center of platter using wooden spatula to pat into a mold. Encircle mold with watercress. Shake salad dressing vigorously and pour to taste over lettuce. Serves 4–6.

WALDORF SALAD

1 cup diced celery	Artificial sweetener equal to 1
2 cups diced apples	tsp. sugar
½ cup broken walnuts	½ cup Mayo 7
2 tbs. lemon juice	lettuce leaves

Dice the celery. Peel, core and dice the apples and sprinkle all with lemon juice and artificial sweetener. Mix in Mayo 7 and half of the walnuts. Serve on a bed of lettuce. Sprinkle with remaining walnuts on top. Serves 4–6.

* We recommend Wagner's
** See Recipe Index

Eggs

CHEESE SOUFFLÉ

1-½ cups fat-free milk
¾ cup water
6 eggs
¼ cup margarine

¼ cup soy flour
1 tsp. salt
Dash cayenne pepper
½ lb. sharp Cheddar

Preheat oven to 300 degrees. In saucepan heat, but do not boil, milk. Separate eggs, putting whites in large bowl, yolks in smaller one. In double boiler, melt margarine, stir in flour, then heated milk, salt, cayenne; cook, stirring, until smooth and thickened. Thinly slice cheese right into sauce. Stir until cheese melts completely and sauce is velvety smooth; remove from heat. With fork, beat egg yolks until well blended. Stir in a little of cheese sauce. Slowly stir this mixture back into rest of cheese sauce. With electric mixer or hand beater, beat egg whites until stiff but not dry. Slowly pour in cheese sauce, folding until no large areas of egg white remain. Pour mixture into *ungreased* 2-qt. casserole up to within ¼ inch of top. (Bake any extra mixture in small *ungreased* casserole.) To form crown, with teaspoon, make shallow path in soufflé mixture about 1 inch in from edge of casserole all the way around. Bake, uncovered, 1¼ hours. *Don't open oven while Soufflé is baking!* Serve at once. Sautéed tomato halves and crisp bacon are nice accompaniments. Makes 6 servings.

POACHED EGGS À LA CHEDDAR

2 eggs
Diet margarine to grease

2 tsp. Cheddar
Dash salt and pepper

Lightly grease nonstick egg poacher with diet margarine. Put in 2 eggs and sprinkle with grated Cheddar, a dash of salt and pepper. Cover pan. Cook over medium heat 3 to 5 minutes. Serve on 2 slices Gluten and Soy Bread.** Serves 1.

** *See Recipe Index*

RASPBERRY OMELET

2 eggs
¼ tsp. salt
2 tbs. milk

1 tbs. sugar-free raspberry
flavoring

Beat eggs, salt, and milk together. Pour into nonstick frying pan. When mixture begins to thicken, pour raspberry syrup on top. Fold into omelet. Serve on warm plate. Serves 1.

SHRIMP OMELET

4 eggs
8 tbs. water or club soda
½ tsp. salt

Dash of pepper
2 tbs. diet margarine
1 cup diced cooked shrimp

Beat the eggs with a wire whisk, add water, salt and pepper. Melt the margarine in a skillet and pour in the egg mixture. Cook over medium heat. When the omelet begins to set, add the diced shrimp. Fold the omelet over from both sides and place on a warm plate to serve. Serves 2.

SPINACH OMELET

4 eggs
½ package frozen chopped
spinach

1 tbs. diet margarine or
butter
Dash salt and pepper

Beat egg yolks and whites in separate mixing bowls with fork or hand mixer. Add salt and pepper to yolks. Then add cooked spinach to yolks and beat. Fold in beaten whites. Grease skillet with diet or regular margarine. Pour in mix; place on burner. When mix is browned turn over omelet with spatula and heat it until omelet appears firm. Slice omelet into 2 portions. Set on plates and serve. Serves 2.

ZUCCHINI OMELET

2 eggs
2 tbs. club soda
Dash of salt and pepper

½ cup sautéed zucchini
Vegetable oil spray for pan

Sauté the zucchini in a little margarine or use leftover stewed zucchini. Break the eggs into a bowl, add the club soda, salt and pepper. Beat well with a wire whisk. Spray a nonstick pan with vegetable oil. Pour in the beaten eggs. When the mixture begins to thicken, add the zucchini. Cook over low heat until the egg mixture is firm. Carefully fold over in thirds. Serve hot. Serves 1.

Meats

BACON OR KOSHER FRY BEEF

1½ ozs. bacon or kosher fry beef, which has less fat

Fry bacon in nonstick pan until crisp. Remove and place on paper towel to let excess fat drain off. Remember, meat weighs as much as an ounce less after cooking. Serve with eggs or use to stuff tomatoes. Serves 1.

BEEF ROULADES

2 lbs. round steak, ¼ inch
½ lb. mushrooms
1 tbs. chopped parsley
¾ cup chopped onion

1 can beef consommé
2 tbs. gluten flour ***
½ cup water
3 tbs. shortening
Salt and pepper

Cut beef into 6 pieces. Flatten with mallet between two sheets of waxed paper. Chop mushroom stems fine. Combine with parsley and onion and season to taste. Place ⅙ of this filling on each piece of meat, roll tightly and tie with string or skewer. Brown on all sides in hot shortening. Add mushroom caps, consommé. Cover and bake in 350-degree oven 1¼ hours. Remove meat from sauce. Thicken sauce with gluten flour dissolved in cold water. Return meat rolls to sauce and serve. Serves 6.

BARBECUED BROILERS

6 broilers, split
1 tsp. salt or salt substitute
⅛ tsp. white pepper
Dash Tabasco
1 tsp. onion juice

½ cup sherry
½ cup sugar-free chili
   sauce ***
½ Papaya Vita ***

Wash broilers and dry on paper towels. Sprinkle with salt or salt substitute and pepper. Bake in oven for half an hour. Baste

*** *Buy in Health Food Store*

66

with sherry occasionally. Combine remaining ingredients to make a sauce and brush over broilers. Barbecue broilers over coals until brown. Serves 8.

CORNED BEEF

5 to 6 lbs. corned brisket of beef
Cold water
Sugar-free mustard

Place meat in large pot. Cover with cold water. Bring to boil, reduce heat and cook slowly for 1 hour. Drain off water, cover with boiling water and cook slowly until tender, 1-½ to 2 hours. Slice thin, place on warm platter and serve with sugar-free mustard. Serves 8–12.

QUICK HASH

1 6-oz. can mushrooms
½ cup whole milk
1 cup diced leftover roast
    beef
½ tsp. onion juice

⅛ tsp. basil
½ tsp. salt
Dash pepper
Chopped parsley for garnish

Drain and chop mushrooms. Place in a saucepan and add milk and onion juice. Heat; then add the roast beef and seasonings. Cook over low heat until most of the liquid is absorbed. Garnish with parsley. Serves 6–8. Serve with a tossed green salad for lunch.

HOT DOGS WITH ARTICHOKE SHELLS

½ lb. artichoke shells **
3 quarts stock (chicken or
    beef)
1 lb. kosher cocktail frank-
    furters

4 tbs. diet margarine
Dash salt
Dash pepper
⅛ tsp. oregano

Boil shells in stock until tender, add salt, pepper and oregano. Boil frankfurters until tender. Combine shells and frankfurters in casserole dish and serve. Serves 4.

** *See Recipe Index*

GRANUAL MEATLOAF

1 lb. ground beef
¼ cup chopped onion
1 tbs. chopped green
  pepper
¼ cup cracked Arti Stix ***
  crumbs
¾ cups soya granuals ***

1 cup canned tomatoes
½ tsp. celery salt
2 tsp. salt
1 beaten egg
½ cup regular or fat-free
  milk
½ tsp. pepper

Mix ingedients well; shape into a loaf and bake in pan oiled with safflower oil at 350 degrees for 1 hour and 15 minutes until brown and well-done. Serves 4–6.

PEPBURGER

1 8-oz. package artichoke
  flour noodles ***
2 lbs. freshly ground
  hamburger
2 cans clear chicken soup
4 cans water
1 tbs. salt
Dash Italian seasoning

1 tsp. hamburger seasoning
¼ tsp. pepper
1 tbs. paprika
1 28-oz. can tomatoes
2 6-oz. cans sugar-free
  tomato sauce ***

Heat the 2 cans chicken soup with 4 cans water to make consommé. Cook artichoke flour noodles in consommé for 7 minutes, or until tender. Drain and salt to taste. Separate meat with fork and brown for 10 minutes in large skillet, over low heat. Drain off fat. Add paprika, salt, pepper, seasonings, tomatoes and tomato sauce. Blend well. Simmer 5 minutes. Add drained noodles and heat all together. Allow to simmer gently uncovered for 5 minutes more. Then serve in large casserole. Serves 4.

*** *Buy in Health Food Store*

PEPPER STEAK

1 top sirloin steak, about 2
   lbs., sliced by butcher
   for pepper steak
2 tbs. safflower oil
3 tbs. soy flour ***
Dash salt
Dash pepper

2 onions, finely chopped
1 10-½-oz. can consommé
¾ lb. mushrooms, sliced
4 green peppers, in large
   slices
1 tbs. minced parsley

Season meat with salt and pepper and rub soy flour into each side. Heat oil in heavy skillet. Sauté onions and peppers separately and then add to meat after browning it on both sides. Pour consommé over meat and bring to a boil. Reduce heat and simmer for a few minutes until tender. Sprinkle with parsley. This can be baked in oven until tender at around 350 degrees. Serves 4.

SPARKLING POT ROAST

4 lbs. breast of beef
Sprinkling salt and pepper
1 beef bouillon cube
1½ cups red wine

½ lb. mushrooms, sliced
⅛ tsp. steak seasoning
1 tbs. minced onions, fresh
   or dried

Place meat in roasting pan. Sprinkle with salt or salt substitute, and pepper. In a small mixing bowl place 1 bouillon cube, ½ cup red wine, the minced onions and mixed herbs seasoning. Stir until bouillon cube is dissolved. Baste or brush pot roast with this mixture. Place pot roast in oven on broil. Turn to brown underside and baste with mixture. When very brown transfer to Dutch oven. Add a cup of red wine and simmer for 30 minutes. Add mushrooms and simmer until mushrooms are tender. Slice and place on platter. Serves 6–8.

*** *Buy in Health Food Store*

SWEET AND SOUR POT ROAST

4–6 lbs. bottom round roast
2 onions, sliced
1-½ cups boiling water
6 bouillon cubes
Dash Kitchen Bouquet

4 ozs. sugar-free chili
  sauce ***
1 bay leaf
6 peppercorns
Pinch thyme

Brown the beef on all sides, combine the other ingredients and brush on the meat. Cover and cook over low heat 3 hours or until meat is fork-tender. Add more water during cooking if necessary. Serves 8–10.

ROAST BEEF AND MUSTARD

4 lbs. rib roast, boned and
  rolled
3-½ tbs. margarine, butter
  or safflower oil

½ cup soup stock
2 tbs. sugar-free
  mustard ***
Salt and pepper to taste

Rub raw meat with mustard. Season with salt and pepper. Heat margarine and pour over meat. Roast in 450-degree oven about 30 minutes. Then reduce heat to 300 degrees and continue to roast 30 minutes longer. Remove meat and trim off fat. Add soup stock to pan. Bring gravy to a boil and serve separately. Serves 6–8. If you wish, use oven thermometer to test for medium, rare or well-done, as desired.

SHISH KEBAB OF BEEF

2 lbs. beef, cubed
12 medium-sized onions, cut
  in half
24 medium-sized mushroom
  caps
2 green squashes, cubed
½ cup dry red wine

3 green peppers, cut up and
  seeded
½ cup vinegar
½ cup safflower oil
1 tsp. salt
⅛ tsp. pepper
Dash ginger

Combine the wine, oil, vinegar, salt, pepper and ginger. Marinate the meat and vegetables in the mixture for 2 to 3 hours. When your fire is ready arrange the meat and vegetables on 12 skewers. Cook over medium fire until the meat is tender. Baste with the marinade from time to time during cooking. Serves 4–6.

*** *Buy in Health Food Store*

SOY AND BEEF BURGER

6 ozs. lean ground beef
3 ozs. soybeans (garlic
   flavored) ***
¼ tsp. seasoned salt

Dash sugar-free Worcestershire sauce ***
Sugar-free catsup ***

Crush the soybeans. Mix with meat, add the salt and Worcestershire sauce. Mix well and shape into 2 patties. Fry in nonstick pan. Turn once. Cook for 4 minutes on each side. Serve with sugar-free catsup. Serves 2.

BARBECUED SPARERIBS

4 lbs. ribs (beef, veal, or
   pork) cut in serving
   pieces
½ cup chopped onions
½ cup sugar-free crushed
   pineapple
½ tsp. nutmeg
1 tbs. sugar-free
   mustard ***

1-½ cups sugar-free tomato
   sauce ***
2 cups chicken broth
½ cup cider vinegar
2 tbs. paprika
1-½ tsp. salt
⅛ tsp. pepper
1 tsp. pickling spice, tied
   in cheesecloth

Sprinkle salt and pepper on the ribs. Place on a rack in roasting pan in a 350-degree oven for 20 minutes. Turn once. Drain off fat. Remove rack. Add remaining ingredients. Bake for 1 hour, basting frequently. Arrange ribs on a warm platter. Strain sauce into a gravy boat and serve with meat. Serves 4–6.

BAKED PARTY STEAK

1 large sirloin steak, 3
   inches thick
½ cup sugar-free chili
   sauce ***
½ cup sugar-free catsup ***
½ tbs. sugar-free Worcestershire sauce ***

1 large onion, chopped
1 lb. mushrooms, sliced thin
1 tsp. salt
¼ cup green pepper, diced or
   sliced thin
⅛ tsp. pepper
4 tbs. melted margarine

Sauté the onion, mushrooms and pepper in margarine until tender. Season with salt and pepper. Remove fat from steak, sprin-

*** *Buy in Health Food Store*

kle with salt and pepper on both sides. Place in roasting pan, cover with chili sauce, catsup and Worcestershire sauce. Let stand at room temperature for 1 hour. Bake in a hot oven (450 degrees) for 45 minutes, or until meat is cooked to suit your taste. *Do not turn the meat.* Slice steak ½-inch thick. Skim the fat from the pan. Mix the mushroom mixture with the juice in the pan. Heat and pour over the meat. Serves 6–8.

EASY STEAK DINNER

2 lbs. potted steak	2 onions, sliced
Pinch salt	2 stalks celery, chopped
Dash pepper	1 8-oz. can peeled tomatoes
¼ cup oat flour ***	1 carrot, sliced

Flatten meat, sprinkle with salt and pepper on each side. Brush flour on *one side only.* Brown meat quickly on each side in a little margarine, brown onions and celery separately. Add onions and celery to meat, add rest of ingredients, including juice of tomatoes. Cook until partly tender. Remove steak, strain gravy and skim off fat. Add a few grains of flour. Return meat to gravy and cook until tender. Add more seasoning according to taste. Serve on platter with gravy over it. Creamed spinach goes well with this dish. Serves 4.

STEAK AND HERBS WITH MUSHROOMS

6 slices sirloin steak, 1-inch thick each	2 tbs. puréed cooked mushrooms **
Salt to taste	1 cup water or soup stock
6 tbs. diet margarine	1 lb. fresh or frozen Italian string beans
1 small onion, chopped	½ lb. fresh mushrooms
Paprika, caraway seeds, marjoram to taste	

Remove bones from meat; pound and salt. Fry gently on both sides in nonstick pan with margarine. Remove meat from pan. Add onion, paprika, caraway seeds, marjoram and puréed mushrooms to margarine used for frying meat. Add water or soup stock and bring to a boil, stirring constantly. Return meat to pan and simmer until tender (about 15 minutes). Add string beans and mushrooms and cook with meat until done. Serves 4–6.

** *See recipe Index for Mushroom Soup Purée*
*** *Buy in Health Food Store*

BAKED FRESH TONGUE

Fresh tongue, weighing 5 to
  6 lbs.
Salt and pepper to taste
Paprika
Gluten flour ***

Diet margarine
1 onion, sliced
1 cup hot water
1 tsp. horseradish

Immerse tongue in boiling water and cook 10 to 15 minutes. Remove from water and pull off skin. Season with salt, pepper and paprika, roll in flour, dot with margarine. Add onion and water. Cover and place in oven at 350 degrees for 2 to 2-½ hours, depending on size of tongue. Brown uncovered for an additional 15 minutes at end. Add horseradish to sauce in pan. Serves 8–10.

BROILERS WITH GRAPES

 4 broiler halves
 2 tbs. margarine or butter
 ½ cup dry sauterne
 4 brown-rice wafers
32 seedless grapes

Salt or salt substitute to
  taste
1 tsp. Italian seasoning
Dash pepper

Place 4 broiler halves in large pan. Sprinkle lightly with salt or salt substitute and Italian seasoning. Crumble 4 brown-rice wafers. Spread around and on broilers. Pour ½ cup dry sauterne over broilers. Let stand for half an hour. Then put pan in 350-degree oven. Bake for 1 hour. Remove from oven. Sprinkle grapes over and around broilers. Return pan to 350-degree oven for 10 minutes. Serve with frozen asparagus, Hollandaise **, and spinach salad. Serves 4.

BROWN 'N BAKE CHICKEN

6 parts of chicken—breasts,
  legs or thighs, according
  to choice

1 or 2 see-thru cooking bags
Paprika to taste
⅛ tsp. white pepper

*** Buy in Gourmet Food Shop

Dressing

¼ cup sugar-free dressing or
our own HG Salad
Dressing **, to which
the following 5 ingredi-
ents have been added:
Garlic steak seasoning *** to
taste

Dash salt
White pepper to taste
½ tsp. garlic peppercorn ***
1 tsp. artificial chili
sauce **

Wash and dry chicken pieces. Pour half of dressing into bowl. Dip each piece of chicken into dressing until well saturated. Sprinkle with paprika. Place each piece into cooking bag so that they lie flat. Close bag and puncture holes in it. Place bag in shallow pan in 350-degree oven for 1 hour. Serve with broccoli on which the remainder of the dressing can be used. Serves 4.

CHICKEN FRICASSEE

2 broilers weighing 2 lbs.
each, cut up
¾ lbs. chopped veal
1 egg
2 stalks celery
3 carrots
8 sprigs parsley
1 large onion
Salt and pepper to taste

1½ tsp. onion salt
1 can clear chicken soup
or 2 cubes of arti-
ficial consommé or 4
cups boiling water
2 tbs. margarine
1 tbs. Kitchen Bouquet
(optional)

Melt margarine in heavy skillet. Brown chicken pieces in margarine. Add salt and pepper and 4 cups of boiling water, chicken soup or 2 chicken cubes. Cut up celery and carrots, onion and parsley. Tie in a cheesecloth. Transfer chicken mixture to 6-quart pot. Add vegetables and stock. Simmer slowly for 45 minutes. Remove vegetables. Put through blender or strainer to liquify. Return to pot with chicken. Add 1 tbs. of Kitchen Bouquet, if desired. Season the veal with onion salt, salt and pepper. Add egg. Use teaspoon to form tiny meatballs. Brown them in skillet and add to chicken. Cook another 15 minutes.

** *See Recipe Index*
*** *Buy in Health Food Store*

Serve with broccoli with Hollandaise Sauce.** Serves 6–8. Tiny whole white onions, cut up carrots, mushroom caps, tomato wedges may be added to the chicken while it cooks. If vegetables are added you may eliminate the broccoli hollandaise and serve Spinach Salad ** on the side.

CHICKEN WITH HAM AND SWISS

4 chicken breasts (whole)
4 slices cooked ham
4 slices Swiss cheese
1 cup white wine

1 tsp. salt
⅛ tsp. pepper
Dash paprika
Watercress for garnish

Bone the chicken breasts and pound with wooden mallet to flatten. Sprinkle with salt and pepper. Pour wine over the chicken and let marinate in refrigerator 4–6 hours. Drain off wine. Place a slice of ham on each piece of chicken, top with a slice of cheese, sprinkle with paprika. Place in a 350-degree oven and bake for 45 minutes. Place on a warm platter, garnish with watercress, and serve. Serves 4.

CHICKEN AND OLIVE MOUSSE

2 envelopes unflavored
    gelatin
½ cup cold water
2-½ cups hot chicken broth
⅛ tsp. garlic powder
1 tsp. onion juice
½ tsp. thyme
1 tsp. dry mustard

Dash cayenne pepper
1 tbs. lemon juice
2 tsp. salt
½ cup sliced black olives
3 cups diced cold chicken
4 egg whites, stiffly beaten
Greens or fresh fruit for
    garnish

Soften gelatin in cold water, add hot chicken broth, and stir until dissolved. Blend in seasonings. Chill until mixture begins to thicken. Fold in the diced chicken and olives. Fold egg whites into the gelatin mixture. Pour into a 2-quart mold. Chill until firm. Unmold onto a serving plate, garnish with crisp greens or fresh fruit in season. Serves 8–10.

** See Recipe Index

CHICKEN ORIENTAL

4 chicken breasts, sliced
1 cup walnuts, coarsely
  chopped
¼ cup safflower oil
1 cup onions, sliced
2-½ cups chicken broth
½ cup celery
¼ cup soy sauce
2 tbs. soy powder ***

2 tbs. salt
Artificial sweetener equal to
  1 tbs. sugar
1 15-oz. can bamboo shoots
1 15-oz. can water chestnuts,
  sliced
2 cups artichoke flour
  shells **

Heat oil in skillet. Add 1 tbs. salt or salt substitute. Toast walnuts in oil for 10 minutes. Remove. Place sliced chicken in the same skillet and cook until brown—about 15 minutes. Remove. Cook onions and celery until golden. Add half chicken broth. Cook until vegetables are tender. In a mixing bowl combine soy powder, remaining chicken broth, soy sauce and seasonings. Pour over vegetables in skillet. Cook until thickened. Add cooked chicken, bamboo shoots and water chestnuts. Mix well. Top with toasted walnuts. Heat thoroughly. Cook artichoke flour shells in chicken broth until tender and serve. Serves 4.

CHICKEN AND SHRIMP

1 3-lb. chicken, cut up
3 small onions
1-½ tsp. salt
¼ tsp. pepper
¼ cup safflower oil
¼ cup parsley flakes

½ cup sherry
1 8-oz. can sugar-free
  tomato sauce ***
1 lb. raw shrimp, cleaned
1 tsp. dried basil

Sprinkle the chicken with salt and pepper, brown in oil in a Dutch oven. Add the other ingredients except the shrimp. Cover and simmer for 45 minutes. Add the shrimp. Turn up the heat and boil for 3 minutes. Place on a hot serving platter. Serves 4–6.

STUFFED CHICKEN BREASTS

4 whole chicken breasts,
  boned
½ tsp. salt
Dash white pepper

1 cup white seedless grapes
  or mushrooms
1 cup dry white wine
Dash paprika

** *See Recipe Index*
*** *Buy in Health Food Store*

Stuffing

1 cup True HG Bread
  crumbs **
½ cup finely chopped
  mushrooms
½ cup finely chopped celery

2 tbs. finely chopped onion
½ cup diet margarine
Salt and pepper to taste
Radish rosettes and turnip
  flowers for garnish

Saute onions, mushrooms and celery in diet margarine. Add breadcrumbs and toss lightly. Wash chicken breasts, dry on paper towel, sprinkle with salt and pepper. Place equal amount of stuffing on each of 4 chicken breasts. Fold in edges and fasten with wooden toothpicks. Sprinkle with paprika. Pour wine into roasting pan with chicken. Roast in 350-degree oven for 1 hour. Fifteen minutes before serving add the grapes or mushrooms. Baste the chicken occasionally with the wine sauce. Serve on a warm platter garnished with radish rosettes and turnip flowers. Serve with string beans and chopped almonds. Serves 4.

ROAST DUCK

1 6-lb. duck
1 cup sugar-free
  applesauce ***

1 tsp. seasoned salt
⅛ tsp. white pepper
Watercress for garnish

Wash the duck and dry with paper towel. Sprinkle inside and out with salt and pepper. Brush inside and out with applesauce. Place on a rack in a roasting pan in 350-degree oven. Cook for 1 hour. Prick occasionally with fork to drain fat from skin. Use baster to drain off fat from pan. Turn the duck on the other side and roast for 1 hour longer. Turn the heat up to 450 degrees during the last 15 minutes if a more golden color is desired. Crisp carefully under broiler for a few minutes on each side. Transfer to a warm platter, garnish with fresh watercress, and serve. Serves 6.

COLD FRESH HAM

1 fresh ham, 5–6 lbs., boned
  and rolled
1 cup sugar-free crushed
  pineapple

1 tsp. rosemary
1 tsp. salt
⅛ tsp. pepper
Fresh parsley, for garnish

** *See Recipe Index*
*** *Buy in Health Food Store*

Sprinkle ham with salt and pepper and rosemary. Cover with crushed pineapple. Place in roasting pan in 325-degree oven. Cook for 4-½ hours. Cool ham. Slice thin and garnish with fresh parsley. Serves 8–10.

HAM CURED IN CIDER

½ ham, smoked, approximately 5 lbs.
3 qts. cider
12 cloves
1 bay leaf
8 black peppercorns

3 stalks celery, cut into pieces
3 medium onions, peeled and sliced
3 carrots, peeled and sliced

Place the ham in a large kettle. Add the seasonings and vegetables. Cover with cider. Bring to a boil, cover and simmer for 2-½ hours. Let cool in the broth. Chill. Slice thin. Serves 8–10.

DEVILED HAM AND CHEESE GELATIN

1 envelope unflavored gelatin
¼ cup cold water
½ cup boiling water
2 cups low-calorie cottage cheese
½ cup crumbled blue cheese
1 tbs. grated onion

½ cup finely diced celery
2 4-½-oz. cans deviled ham
Lettuce leaves
Our HG Salad Dressing **
Salt and pepper to taste

Soften gelatin in cold water, add boiling water and stir until dissolved. Chill until slightly thickened. Mix in the cottage cheese, blue cheese, salt and pepper, onion and celery. Pour half the mixture into a 1-½-qt. ring mold. Chill until set. Spread a layer of deviled ham evenly over the cheese. Spoon the remaining cheese mixture over the ham. Chill until set. Unmold on platter, surround with lettuce leaves. Serve with dressing. Serves 4–6.

** *See Recipe Index*

GROUND HAM AND PINEAPPLE

1 cup cooked ham, ground   2 tbs. Mayo 7
1 tsp. sugar-free mustard ***   4 slices sugar-free pineapple

Combine the first three ingredients. Place pineapple slices in shallow baking pan. Top with the ham mixture and bake in a 350-degree oven for 15 minutes. Serves 4.

HAM AND CHICKEN IN WINE

6 large chicken breasts   1 cup dry white wine
6 slices ham   Dash salt
6 slices Swiss cheese without   Dash pepper
  holes   Watercress for garnish

Marinate chicken in wine for 30 minutes, place in shallow roasting pan, and add seasonings. Place 1 slice of ham and 1 slice of Swiss cheese over each chicken breast. Put in 350-degree oven for 30 to 45 minutes. Before serving, garnish with clusters of crisp watercress. Serves 4–6.

Variations:

HAM AND CORNED BEEF IN WINE

Substitute 6-inch-thick slices boiled lean corned beef for chicken breasts.

HAM AND VEAL CUTLETS IN WINE

Substitute 6-inch-thick veal chops for chicken breasts.

MUSHROOMS AND HAM

1 lb. fresh mushrooms   2 tbs. soy flour ***
2 tbs. lemon juice   1 tsp. salt
2 tbs. margarine   ⅛ tsp. pepper
½ cup minced onion   ¼ tsp. nutmeg
2 cups minced ham   1-½ cups yogurt
Chopped parsley   2 tbs. sherry

*** *Buy in Health Food Store*

79

Select small mushrooms; leave them whole. Wash and wipe dry on paper towel; sprinkle with lemon juice. Place in a baking dish with melted margarine, onion and parsley. Bake in a 350-degree oven for 10 minutes. Mix in the ham. In a saucepan mix the soy flour, salt, pepper, nutmeg and yogurt. Stir until thickened. Add the sherry and mix with the mushrooms and ham. Serve with De Boles noodles ***. Serves 4.

ROAST FRESH HAM

1 5-lb. fresh ham	1 cup water
16 whole cloves	1-½ cups dry white wine
2 bay leaves	1-½ tsp. salt
1 tbs. caraway seeds	½ tsp. pepper
1 clove garlic	

Remove skin from ham. Score fat in two directions. Rub meat on all sides with salt, pepper, caraway seeds and garlic. Stick cloves into fat on meat. Lay bay leaves on top. Place in a roasting pan and pour water and wine over ham. Roast in a 325-degree oven for 4-½ to 5 hours. Baste from time to time with pan juices. Serves 8–10.

STUFFED HAM SLICES

2 center-cut, fully cooked ham slices, one inch thick	1 cup chopped celery leaves
	½ tsp. nutmeg
	Dash cayenne
12 cloves	1 tsp. salt
½ lb. fresh spinach	⅛ tsp. pepper
1 cup chopped green scallions	

Stud cloves in fat on each ham slice. Mix the remaining ingredients and place on top of ham slices. Cover with remaining slice and fasten with skewers. Bake in 325-degree oven for 2 hours. Place on a warm platter and serve. Serves 6–8.

LAMB SHISH KEBAB

2-½ lbs. lamb, cubed
12 medium-sized onions
4 green peppers
3 tomatoes

1 cup dry red wine
½ cup safflower oil
Salt and pepper to taste
12 skewers, 15 inches long

Combine wine, oil, salt and pepper. Marinate the meat in this mixture for 2 hours. Cut the onions in half, cut peppers into pieces. Remove seeds and fiber. Add to the meat and mix to coat with marinade. Cut tomatoes into wedges. Arrange on skewers. Cook over charcoal until meat is tender. Baste occasionally with the marinade during cooking. Serve hot with a tossed salad and Our HG Salad Dressing **. Serves 4–6.

RAGOUT OF LAMB

3 lbs. leg of lamb, boned, cut
   in 1-inch cubes
Gluten flour ***
Salt and pepper
3 tbs. safflower oil
1 small white onion, minced

1-½ cups strong, hot chicken
   broth
½ cup sherry
2 tbs. lemon juice, fresh
2 tbs. parsley, chopped
   fine

Trim off all visible fat and skin from lamb. Dredge cubes in gluten flour, salt and pepper. Heat oil in frying pan and sauté lamb until lightly browned. Add onion, pour over broth and sherry, heat to bubbling, cover and reduce heat. Simmer about 1 hour. Add lemon juice and parsley, stir, bring to boil and serve. Add juice and parsley just before serving. Serves 6.

MIXED GRILL

3 slices leg of veal, cut
   ¼ inch thick
½ lb. salami, sliced
½ lb. bologna, sliced
¼ cup True HG Bread
   crumbs **
½ cup diced onions
2 tbs. chopped parsley

1 tsp. dried basil
6 hard-boiled eggs
¼ cup safflower oil
½ tsp. salt
⅛ tsp. pepper
6 slices bacon
2 cups sugar-free tomato
   sauce ***

Have the bone removed from the veal but leave each slice whole. Pound the cutlets very thin. On a large sheet of waxed paper

** *See Recipe Index*
*** *Buy in Health Food Store*

arrange the slices side by side the long way so that they overlap slightly. Pound the overlapping edges to press them together. On the veal arrange overlapping slices of salami. Top with rows of bologna, sprinkle with breadcrumbs and diced onions, parsley and basil. Place a row of hard-boiled eggs down the center, sprinkle with oil, salt and pepper; carefully roll up in the paper as for a jelly roll. Make sure the eggs stay in place in the center. Remove the paper. Tie the meat firmly in 5 or 6 places. Place in a baking dish and top with bacon slices. Pour tomato sauce over all. Bake in 350-degree oven for 1 hour, basting occasionally with the tomato sauce. Remove to a hot platter and slice. Serve with Lange's Mixed Vegetable Macaroni *** and a green salad. Serves 4–6.

PORK CHOPS AND CHEESE

6 pork chops, 1-inch thick	1 clove garlic, minced
2 tsp. salt	2 tbs. lemon juice
½ tsp. pepper	2 cups grated cheddar cheese

Trim fat from chops. Rub with garlic, salt and pepper. Sprinkle with lemon juice. Place in baking dish in a 350-degree oven for 35 minutes. Sprinkle with cheese and bake 20 minutes longer. Serves 6.

PORK CHOPS WITH OLIVES

6 pork chops, 1-inch thick	2 cups fresh tomatoes,
½ cup oat flour ***	peeled and chopped
2 tsp. salt	¾ cup dry white wine
½ tsp. pepper	2 hard-boiled eggs, chopped
¼ cup safflower oil	½ cup stuffed olives, sliced
1 cup onions, sliced	

Mix 1 tsp. salt and ¼ tsp. pepper with oat flour. Trim fat from chops and dip them in flour. Brown on both sides in hot oil. Remove chops. Sauté the onions for 5 minutes; add the tomatoes and remaining salt and pepper. Cook over low heat for 10 minutes. Stir in the wine and return the chops to pan. Baste well with the sauce. Cover and cook in a 350-degree oven for 1 hour. Remove the cover, sprinkle with egg and olives and cook 10 minutes longer. Serves 6.

*** *Buy in Health Food Store*

PORK CHOPS AND SOUR CREAM

6 pork chops, 1-inch thick
¼ cup safflower oil
1 tsp. salt
½ tsp. pepper

1 cup sour cream or sour
   cream substitute
2 tsp. capers
3 tbs. dill pickle, diced

Season chops with salt and pepper. Brown in oil on both sides. Add the sour cream and cover. Cook over low heat for 45 minutes. Turn chops a few times. Add more sour cream if necessary. Stir in capers and pickle. Serves 6.

BAKED VEAL CHOPS

6 7-oz. veal chops with bone
   (each loses 1 oz. in
   cooking)
3 tomatoes
Juice of 1½ lemons
6 white onions
1 tsp. garlic bread seasoning

Pinch Italian seasoning
 2 tsp. salt
Dash paprika
¼ green pepper
Parsley for garnish
Radish rosettes for garnish

Marinate chops in lemon juice and garlic seasoning for at least 30 minutes. Then place chops in baking pan. Cut up, but do not mince, tomatoes, onions, and green pepper. Mix with ½ tsp. salt and pinch Italian seasoning. Then spread mix over and around chops. Add pinch pepper and sprinkle with remaining salt. Bake in a 350-degree oven for 50 minutes. Garnish with parsley and radish rosettes. Serves 6.

BREADED VEAL CUTLET

4 veal cutlets, weighing 3 ozs.
   each
2 eggs, beaten
1 cup Arti Stix *** crumbs

1 tsp. salt
⅛ tsp. pepper
⅛ tsp. thyme
¼ cup safflower oil

Combine the Arti Stix crumbs, salt, pepper and thyme. Dip the cutlets in beaten egg, then in crumbs. Coat well. Fry in hot oil until golden brown. Serves 4 for breakfast or 2 for dinner.

COUNTRY CHICKS

1 lb. veal, cut into 1-inch
    cubes
1 lb. lean pork, cut into
    1-inch cubes
12 medium-sized mushroom
    caps
1 egg, beaten

1 tsp. salt
⅛ tsp. pepper
2 tbs. oat flour ***
½ cup Arti Stix,***
    crumbled
12 15-inch-long skewers

Sprinkle the meat with salt and pepper. Dip in oat flour, then in beaten egg, then in crumbs. Arrange on skewers as follows: 1 cube of pork, 1 cube of veal, 2 mushroom caps. Repeat layers until skewers are full. Cook over charcoal fire until the meat is tender. Serves 6–8.

CREAMED VEAL

3 lbs. veal shoulder
Salt to taste
6 tbs. butter or diet mar-
    garine
½ cup soup stock or more
Sliced apples—about 6

½ head cauliflower, sep-
    arated into flowerets
    and cooked in salted
    water
Artificial sweetener to taste

White Sauce

3 tbs. butter or margarine
3 tbs. oat or gluten flour ***

¼ tsp. salt
½-1 cup soup stock

Wash, skin and cut meat into 1-inch cubes. Add salt. Brown slightly in butter or margarine. Add soup stock as needed and simmer until tender, 1 hour or more. Prepare white sauce: Melt butter or margarine, add flour and stir until smooth. Add soup stock and salt and stir constantly until thickened. Add sauce to meat and stir well. Bake apple slices until tender in artificial sweetener. Then add apples and cooked cauliflower to meat mixture and serve. Serves 6.

*** *Buy in Health Food Store*

LEFTOVER ROAST VEAL GOULASH

2-¾ lbs. leftover roast veal
  1 cup leftover gravy
  5 tbs. safflower oil
  2 medium onions, sliced
  1 tbs. vinegar
Caraway seeds to taste
Marjoram to taste
Sprinkling of seasoned salt
    or salt substitute

1-½ cups water or stock
  1 tsp. gluten flour ***
1-½ cups canned stringbeans
  ½ cup frozen baby limas
  1 stalk celery, cut in half
  1 chopped sour pickle
  2 tbs. diet margarine
  1 tsp. paprika

Cut meat into large chunks. Heat oil, add sliced onions and brown gently until golden in color. Add meat. Add vinegar, caraway seeds, marjoram and seasoned salt or salt substitute. Add 1 cup water or soup stock gradually. Simmer on low flame for 30 minutes. Add flour and boil a few minutes. Then add vegetables and chopped pickle. Simmer mixture for 30 minutes more. In separate small pan heat paprika in 2 tbs. margarine. Add remaining soup stock and water and gravy. Then pour whole over the goulash when ready to serve. Serves 4.

SHISH KEBAB OF VEAL

  2 lbs. veal, cubed
24 medium-sized mushroom
    caps
12 medium-sized onions, cut
    in half
  3 green peppers, cut into
    quarters and seeded
  ½ cup dry white wine

  ½ cup dry red wine
  ¼ cup safflower oil
  1 tsp. oregano
  1 tsp. salt
  ⅛ tsp. pepper
24 cubes yellow turnips,
    parboiled
12 15-inch-long skewers

Make a marinade of the wines, oil, salt, pepper and oregano. Place meat and vegetables in a large bowl. Pour the marinade over the mixture and put in the refrigerator for 3 to 4 hours. When your fire is ready, arrange the meat and vegetables on 12 long skewers. Cook over medium fire until the meat is tender. Serves 4–6.

*** *Buy in Health Food Store*

STUFFED GREEN PEPPERS

4 medium-sized green
  peppers
1 cup chopped cooked
  veal

½ cup chopped sautéed mushrooms
2 tbs. safflower oil
½ tsp. salt

Cook the peppers in boiling, salted water for 5 minutes. Drain, sprinkle with salt, cool. Combine the other ingredients. Remove cores from the peppers, fill with the meat mixture. Bake in a 350-degree oven for 40 minutes. This is a good luncheon dish. Serves 4.

VEAL AND ALMONDS

1-½ lbs. veal
1 tsp. salt
½ cup Arti Stix,***
  crumbled

2 tbs. oat flour ***
2 tbs. margarine
½ cup sliced almonds
1 egg, beaten

Cook the veal in salted water until tender (about 30 minutes). Drain and save the liquid. Chop the meat fine and add to 1 cup of the liquid. Mix the meat mixture with the Arti Stix crumbs, flour, margarine and almonds. Shape into patties. Dip in beaten egg and a little Arti Stix crumbs. Sauté in melted margarine until browned, turning once. Serves 6.

VEAL BIRDS

1-½ lbs. veal cutlets
¼ lb. ground veal
½ cup Arti Stix ***
  crumbs
1 tsp. salt

⅛ tsp. pepper
1 egg, beaten
½ cup soy flour ***
½ cup safflower oil
Light cream

Pound the veal very thin, cut into 2 × 4-inch pieces. Mix the ground veal, Arti Stix crumbs, salt, pepper, and egg. Spread on the pieces of veal. Roll up and fasten with toothpicks. Sprinkle with salt and pepper, roll in soy flour. Cook in hot oil until browned. Add enough light cream to half-cover the meat. Cover and cook in a 350-degree oven until tender, about 1 hour. Serves 4–6.

*** *Buy in Health Food Store*

VEAL CHOPS AND CHEESE

4 veal chops, 1-½ inches
    thick
1 tbs. safflower oil
1 tsp. salt

⅛ tsp. pepper
¼ tsp. sage
4 slices American cheese

Place the chops in a shallow pan. Sprinkle with salt, pepper, sage and oil. Place under the broiler for 10 minutes, turn, sprinkle again with seasonings and oil and top each chop with a slice of cheese. Continue to cook until cheese melts. Serves 4.

VEAL CUTLETS WITH EGGPLANT

2 lbs. veal cutlets
1 medium eggplant, sliced
1 onion, sliced
1 cup diced green pepper
8 black olives
¾ cup safflower oil
1 tsp. salt

⅛ tsp. pepper
½ tsp. oregano
1 cup sugar-free tomato
    sauce ***
½ lb. mushrooms, sliced
    (optional)

Brown the meat on both sides in hot oil. In a 1-½-qt. casserole, arrange layers of eggplant, veal, onions, green pepper and mushrooms, if used. Sprinkle with salt, pepper and oregano. Pour tomato sauce over mixture and bake in a 350-degree oven for 1 to 1-½ hours. Serves 6.

VEAL CUTLETS AU VIN

1-½ lbs. veal cutlets
1 tbs. safflower oil
1 tbs. chopped onion
2 tbs. chopped ham
1 tsp. chopped parsley

¼ cup dry white wine
½ cup water
1 tsp. salt
⅛ tsp. pepper

Heat the oil in skillet, add the veal and cook for 10 minutes, turning once to brown. Add the onion, ham and parsley. Cover and cook slowly for 15 to 20 minutes. Add the wine and cook 10 minutes longer. Transfer the meat to a hot platter. Add the water, salt and pepper to the pan, and bring to a boil. Pour over the meat and serve. Serves 4.

*** *Buy in Health Food Store*

VEAL WITH EGGS

2 lbs. veal cutlets, pounded thin
1 cup Arti Stix *** crumbs
1 tsp. salt

⅛ tsp. pepper
2 eggs, beaten
¾ cup safflower oil
6 fried eggs

Roll the Arti Stix into crumbs. Mix in salt and pepper. Dip the veal in crumbs, then in beaten egg, and again in crumbs. Sauté in hot oil until tender. Place a fried egg on each cutlet and serve. Serves 6.

VEAL FRICANDEAU

3 lbs. veal shoulder or piece cut from upper part of leg

Dash salt
3 oz. ham, cut into strips
½ cup stock

Sauce

1 cup sour cream or sour cream substitute
4 egg yolks
¾ cup grated cheddar
1 tbs. Arti Stix,*** crumbled

1 tbs. melted butter or margarine
1 tbs. freshly grated Parmesan

Skin and salt meat. Cover with strips of ham. Simmer in deep pan with soup for 1-¼ hours. Cut meat into thin slices. Arrange meat and ham in ovenproof dish. Prepare sauce: Beat sour cream, egg yolks and cheddar in double boiler until thick. Sprinkle with Arti Stix crumbs. Pour over meat. Pour melted margarine or butter on top. Sprinkle with grated Parmesan and roast in hot oven 5–10 minutes, until slightly crusty. Serves 6.

*** *Buy in Health Food Store*

VEAL MARSALA

2 lbs. veal cutlets
¼ cup oat flour ***
1 tsp. salt
⅛ tsp. white pepper
⅓ cup diet margarine,
  melted

¾ lb. fresh mushrooms,
  sliced
1 chicken bouillon cube
½ cup boiling water
½ cup Marsala

Coat the meat with flour, season with salt and pepper. Brown the meat in hot melted margarine on both sides. Remove from pan, add mushrooms to pan and cook for a few minutes. Pour in the water, add the chicken bouillon cube and Marsala. Return the meat to pan, cook until bubbling, and serve. Serves 4.

VEAL AND MUSHROOMS

1-½ lbs. veal cutlets, cut in
    3-inch pieces
1 lb. mushrooms, sliced
2 tbs. safflower oil

1 tsp. salt
⅛ tsp. pepper
1 cup light cream

Sprinkle veal pieces with salt and pepper and sauté 3 or 4 pieces of veal at a time with some sliced mushrooms. When all the veal is cooked, return to pan. Add the cream, heat just under boiling point (*do not boil*), and serve. Serves 4–6.

VEAL ROAST I

4 lbs. boneless veal roast
½ tsp. salt
⅛ tsp. pepper
1 tsp. paprika

Dash garlic powder
1 can chicken bouillon
2 tbs. sherry

Sprinkle the meat with salt, pepper and garlic powder. Brown on all sides. (This may be done either on top of the stove or under the broiler.) Pour chicken bouillon over roast and sprinkle with paprika. Roast in 350-degree oven for 1-½ hours. Remove meat and slice. Add the sherry to the liquid in pan and serve as sauce with meat. Serve 6–8.

*** *Buy in Health Food Store*

VEAL ROAST II

6 lbs. boneless veal roast　　　1 tsp. salt
2 cups sugar-free tomato　　　⅛ tsp. white pepper
　　juice　　　　　　　　　　½ tsp. paprika
1 can chicken bouillon　　　　½ cup light cream
1 can water

Sprinkle meat with salt and pepper. Brown on all sides. Place in roasting pan. Sprinkle with paprika. Pour the tomato juice over the meat and cook in a 350-degree oven for 45 minutes. Combine bouillon with the water and pour over meat. Continue to cook for 1 hour longer. Baste occasionally with pan juices. When meat is done remove to serving platter. Add light cream to the juice in the pan and heat until ready to bubble. Serve as sauce with veal. Serves 8.

VEAL WITH SALMON

4 lbs. veal shoulder　　　　　2 egg yolks
1 cup white wine　　　　　　½ cup safflower oil
3 sprigs parsley　　　　　　½ tsp. salt
2 sprigs fresh dill　　　　　　⅛ tsp. pepper
2 7-oz. cans salmon

Have the butcher bone, roll and tie the veal. Place meat in deep casserole with a tight cover, add the wine, parsley, dill, salmon, salt and pepper. Cover and place in a 350-degree oven for 3 hours. Let casserole cool, then place in refrigerator to chill. Purée the salmon and juices in electric blender. Beat the egg yolks until light and lemon-colored. Gradually add oil. Slowly beat in the salmon mixture. Cut the veal into thin slices and arrange on platter. Pour the sauce over. Serves 8–10.

VEAL SCALLOPINE WITH SHERRY

2 lbs. veal cutlets　　　　　½ tsp. pepper
½ cup oat flour ***　　　　　½ cup safflower oil
1-½ tsp. salt　　　　　　　½ cup Marsala

Pound the cutlets thin, cut into pieces and roll in flour. Sprinkle with salt and pepper. Cook in hot oil until browned and tender. Add the wine and bring to boil. Place on a warm platter and serve. Serves 6.

*** *Buy in Health Food Store*

VEAL STEW

2 lbs. veal shoulder
2 tbs. diet margarine
12 small white onions
1 lb. stringbeans
3 stalks celery

1 small yellow turnip
4 large tomatoes
4 cups boiling water
Salt and pepper to taste
3 tbs. gluten flour ***

Cut veal into 1-½-inch cubes, brown on all sides in hot margarine. Prepare vegetables for cooking. Leave onions and stringbeans whole. Cut celery into 2-inch pieces. Peel turnip and cut into 1-inch cubes. Peel tomatoes and cut into quarters. Add the vegetables, salt and pepper to the meat, add 4 cups boiling water, cover and cook slowly until meat is tender. Remove meat and vegetables to a serving dish. Thicken the liquid with a paste made of 3 tbs. gluten flour and cold water. Pour gravy over meat or serve separately. Serves 6–8.

VEAL-STUFFED ZUCCHINI

4 medium-size zucchini
2 qts. boiling, salted water
3 tbs. safflower oil
¾ lb. ground veal
2 tbs. chopped onion
2 eggs, beaten

¼ cup freshly grated Parmesan
1 tsp. salt
⅛ tsp. pepper
¼ tsp. marjoram
1 tsp. chopped parsley

Cook the zucchini in boiling, salted water until tender. Drain and cool. Cut in half lengthwise. Scoop out pulp and mash it. Heat the oil in a skillet. Cook the onion until soft, add the salt, pepper and marjoram. Add the ground veal. Cook until browned. Mix the zucchini pulp with the meat mixture, cool slightly and add the eggs and Parmesan. Mix well. Stuff the zucchini shells with the meat mixture. Sprinkle with chopped parsley. Bake in a 350-degree oven for 30 minutes. Serves 6–8.

*** *Buy in Health Food Store*

WIENER SCHNITZEL

2 lbs. veal cutlets
½ cup oat flour ***
1 cup Arti Stix *** (rolled
    into crumbs)
½ cup melted diet margarine
    or butter

2 eggs beaten
Juice of 1 lemon
3 tbs. chopped parsley
1 tsp. salt
¼ tsp. pepper
¼ marjoram

Combine flour, salt and pepper. Cut the veal into 1-½ inch pieces. Dip each piece in flour, then dip in beaten eggs and finally in crumbs. Melt half the margarine in skillet. Brown the meat on both sides for about 5 minutes or until tender. Place on a hot platter. Add the remaining margarine to the skillet and allow to brown. Add the parsley, lemon juice, and marjoram. Pour over the veal and serve. Serves 6.

*** *Buy in Health Food Store*

Fish

BROILED HADDOCK

2 lbs. haddock filets
Salt and pepper to taste
½ cup True HG Bread-
crumbs **

4 tbs. diet margarine
12 fresh grapefruit sections
¼ tsp. crumbled thyme

Wipe filets dry with paper towel. Sprinkle both sides with salt and pepper. Place in a shallow nonstick baking pan. Mix the breadcrumbs with ½ of melted margarine and thyme and sprinkle over fish, top with grapefruit sections. Brush with remaining melted margarine. Broil from 25–30 minutes, or until fish is flaky. Serves 4.

CURRIED HAKE

3 onions, chopped
1 small green pepper,
chopped
1 tbs. curry powder
¼ cup diet margarine

4 whole cloves
1 stick cinnamon
½ cup undiluted evap-
orated milk
1-½ lbs. hake filets, cubed

Cook the onion, green pepper and curry powder in margarine for 5 minutes. Add the cloves, cinnamon, milk and fish. Add salt to taste and simmer for 15 minutes. Serves 2–4. Serve with baked potato, asparagus and tossed green salad. Note: Do not eat any bread the day you have this meal. The baked potato is your starch for the day.

BARBECUED HALIBUT STEAKS

4 halibut steaks weighing
about ¾ of a pound each
(be sure to ask for *male*
halibut steaks)
6 peppercorns
Sea salt ***

½ cup lemon juice
Diet or regular margarine or
butter
Dash garlic salt
1 tsp. seafood seasoning
Parsley or watercress for
garnish

** *See Recipe Index*
*** *Buy in Health Food Store*

Marinate fish in lemon juice. Refrigerate for 1 or 2 hours. Start your fire early enough to allow coals to turn white before cooking. Cover grill with silver foil. Set fish on grill. Baste with lemon juice and butter mixed with garlic salt. Sprinkle liberally with sea salt, peppercorns, and seafood seasoning. When fish becomes tender, poke holes with fork in silver foil, around and between steaks. Let cook a few minutes longer. Set fish on platter and garnish with parsley or watercress. Serves 4.

DEVILED HALIBUT STEAKS

4 medium-sized halibut
   steaks (be sure to ask for
   male halibut steaks)
2 tbs. prepared, sugar-free
   mustard ***

2 tbs. sugar-free chili
   sauce ***
2 tbs. prepared horseradish
1 tsp. salt

Wipe fish with paper towel and place in shallow pan. Mix the other ingredients and spread half of it over the fish. Place in the broiler and broil for 8 minutes. Turn the fish, spread with remaining sauce and cook 8–10 minutes longer. Place on a warm platter. Garnish with lemon wedges. Serves 4.

HALIBUT WITH DILL

4 medium-sized halibut
   steaks (be sure to ask for
   male halibut steaks)
Salt or salt substitute
Black pepper, if desired

3 tbs. sour cream
⅛ tsp. dry mustard
1/16 tsp. hot curry powder
12 sprigs fresh dill
¼ tsp. Chinese Five Spice *

Place halibut in shallow pan. Combine rest of ingredients except for dill. Brush over the fish. Top with dill. Place in 350-degree oven and bake for 20 minutes. Place under broiler until top becomes brown. Garnish with lemon wedges. Serves 4.

HALIBUT MOUSSE

1 lb. halibut, cooked
3 egg whites
1 cup evaporated milk
Pan of ice water

Pan of hot water
1 tsp. salt
⅛ tsp. pepper
⅛ tsp. celery salt

* *Buy in Oriental Food Shop*
*** *Buy in Health Food Store*

Skin the fish. Put through a food chopper, using the fine blade. Place fish in a bowl, set the bowl in a pan of ice water. Slowly add the egg whites, beat with a wire whisk until the mixture is smooth. Slowly stir in remaining ingredients. Place in refrigerator for 1 hour. Grease a 1-½-qt. mold. Pour in the mixture, set in a pan of hot water and bake in a 350-degree oven until firm (35 to 45 minutes). Serves 4–6.

HALIBUT WITH PEANUTS

6 halibut steaks or 6 red
   snapper filets
1 cup dry roasted peanuts,
   preferably unsalted
1 cup dry white wine

Salt to taste
Regular or diet margarine or
   butter
Italian seasoning to taste

Put fish in shallow pan. Sprinkle with salt or salt substitute and Italian seasoning. Then pour white wine over the fish. Put dabs of margarine or butter over fish. After marinating for several hours, place pan in 350-degree oven for half hour. Remove pan and spread nuts over fish. Turn oven up to broil and return pan to oven for 10 to 15 minutes. Serves 6.

HALIBUT WITH MUSTARD SAUCE

4 medium-sized halibut
   steaks (be sure to ask
   for *male* halibut steaks)
¼ cup diet margarine
¼ cup soy or gluten flour ***
½ tsp. sugar-free chili
   sauce ***

½ tsp. powdered mustard
½ tsp. salt
⅛ tsp. white pepper
2 cups milk
1 tbs. minced chives
Dash paprika

Wipe fish with paper towel. Poach in seasoned simmering water to cover until fish flakes. (See recipe for Halibut Steaks with Curry Sauce. Drain and leave fish in covered pan. Melt the margarine and blend in the flour and seasonings; add milk. (You may use 1 cup of milk and 1 cup of the fish stock, if desired.) Cook until thickened. Put fish on a hot platter and pour sauce over. Sprinkle with chives and paprika. Serves 4.

*** *Buy in Health Food Store*

HALIBUT RING

2-½ lbs. halibut
1 bay leaf
3 whole cloves
2 slices lemon
2 tsp. seafood seasoning
⅛ tsp. white pepper
½ tsp. paprika
1 tbs. chopped parsley

1 tsp. Italian seasoning
½ tsp. dried dill
2 cups whole milk
6 egg yolks, beaten
6 egg whites, beaten
½ tsp tarragon leaves
Parsley for garnish

Poach fish in boiling salted water with 1 bay leaf, 3 cloves, and 2 slices lemon. Skin, bone and flake fish. Add seasonings and mix. Add beaten egg yolks. Continue to mix. Gradually add 2 cups milk. Fold in stiffly beaten egg whites. Grease 1-½-qt. fish-shaped or ring mold. Spoon in mixture. Place mold into pan of water and bake in 350-degree oven for about 50 to 60 minutes, until firm. Unmold onto heated platter. Garnish with fresh parsley and serve with Mushroom Sauce ** or Grape and White Wine Sauce **. Serves 6–8.

HALIBUT STEAKS WITH CURRY SAUCE

4 medium-sized halibut
    steaks (be sure to ask for
    male halibut steaks)
2 slices onion
2 parsley sprigs
1 celery top

½ tsp. salt
4 peppercorns or ⅛ tsp.
    ground pepper
½ lemon
Boiling water

Place the fish in poacher. Cover with boiling water, add remaining ingredients. Cover and simmer for 15 minutes until the fish is tender. Place fish on hot platter. Reserve broth for curry sauce (see following recipe). Serves 4–6.

Curry Sauce

4 tbs. diet margarine
½ onion, grated
2 tsp. soy or gluten flour ***
3–4 tsp. curry powder

½ tsp. salt
1-½ cups fish stock
¼ cup undiluted evaporated
    milk

Cook the onion in margarine until tender. Blend in flour and seasonings. Slowly add fish stock. Cook until thickened, stirring constantly. Add milk before serving. Pour over fish steaks or serve separately.

** *See Recipe Index*
*** *Buy in Health Food Store*

BROILED LOBSTER

4 freshly boiled lobsters	½ tsp. white pepper
1 cup melted diet margarine	Paprika
2 tsp. salt	Lemon wedges

Split and clean the lobsters. Place meat side up on a broiler pan. Brush generously with margarine. Sprinkle with salt, pepper, and paprika. Broil under medium heat until lobster is heated through. Garnish with lemon wedges and serve. Serves 4.

A Cheerful Tail . . .

SPICY BROILED LOBSTER

3 lbs. shelled lobster tails, cooked and cut into chunks	1 tbs. Dijon or other sugar-free mustard
1 small finely diced green pepper	½ tsp. white pepper
	Dash seasoned salt
1 tbs. salt	2 eggs
	1 cup Mayo 7

Beat eggs and combine with Mayo 7, green pepper and seasonings. Fold in lobster meat. Put mixture in shells or ramekins. Top with Mayo 7 and sprinkle with paprika. Broil for a few minutes, until delicately browned. Serves 8–10.

BOILED SALMON WITH PEPPERCORNS

2 lbs. fresh salmon wrapped in vegetable parchment paper	For garnish:
	Lettuce leaves
A few cloves, bay leaves, and peppercorns	Tomato wedges
	Cucumber
Liberal sprinkling of mono-sodium glutamate	Radish rosettes
	Deviled eggs
1 tsp. salt	Dressings:
1 white onion	Cold Hollandaise **
Juice of one lemon, and half of rind	Horseradish sauce
	Yogurt

Put salmon in pot, add water but do not let it cover fish. Add rest of ingredients and leave one-half lemon rind in water. Cover

** *See Recipe Index*

pot. Bring to boil, then let it simmer for 25 minutes. Remove fish onto a deep platter and remove paper. Pour liquid over rest of ingredients and leave one-half lemon rind in water. Cover fish and let it chill in refrigerator for at least 3 hours. Serves 4–5. When ready to serve: Garnish a platter with lettuce leaves, tomato wedges, cucumber, radish rosettes, and deviled eggs. Place salmon on platter. For a dressing use cold Hollandaise ** or a horseradish sauce or just plain yogurt.

FRESH SALMON CHABLIS

2 medium-sized salmon
    steaks
Diet margarine
⅛ tsp. salt or salt substitute
Dash pepper

4 oz. dry Chablis
1 tbs. freshly chopped
    parsley
Dash seasoned salt

Rub salmon with margarine, salt and pepper. Broil for 15 minutes until brown. Turn oven on to Bake at 450 degrees for 10 minutes. Put parsley flakes in wine and a dash of seasoned salt. Pour very, very slowly over fish so that it seeps through. Let it cook another 5 minutes. Garnish with lemon wedges and watercress. Serve with creamed spinach. Serves 4.

A Delicious Salmon Barbecue . . .

SAUMON AVEC POISSONADE
AU CHARBON DE BOIS

2 2-¼-lb. salmon steaks
Juice of 3 large fresh lemons
    or 6 small ones
1 bay leaf, crumbled
Poissonade *** (thyme, basil,
    sarriette, green anise,
    and flowers of lavender)
    in the amount that suits
    taste

Sprinkling seafood seasoning
1 tbs. margarine or butter
1 tsp. chives
Sea salt ***
Black pepper to taste
Paprika
Watercress for garnish

Clean fish steaks and dry with paper towel. Pour lemon juice carefully over the fish. Sprinkle with Poissonade to taste, sea salt, black pepper and a pinch of crumbled bay leaves. Set in

*** *Buy in Health Food Store*

refrigerator and allow to chill and marinate for 1–2 hours. When your fire is ready put the steaks on grill over silver foil. Broil for 10 minutes and then turn steaks over—once only. Dab a little margarine or butter over fish. Sprinkle with paprika, seafood seasoning, sea salt, black pepper and lastly chives. Cook until fish is tender, but not soft. Set on platter and garnish with watercress. Serves 6.

SALMON RING

2 lbs. salmon (cooked or canned)	½ tsp. celery salt
	½ tsp. salt
6 egg yolks	Dash of pepper
6 egg whites, stiffly beaten	3 tbs. soy flour ***
1 tsp. onion juice	1 cup fish stock or water

Put fish through food chopper and place in large mixing bowl. Beat egg yolks well and add to fish. Add seasonings, fish stock and soy flour. Beat egg whites until stiff. Fold into the fish mixture. Grease well with low-calorie margarine or butter. Place in a 2-quart ring mold. Spoon the mixture into mold. Set mold in a pan of hot water and bake in 350-degree oven until firm. Serves 6–8.

SALMON AND SOYBEANS

4 slices salmon steaks	2 apples, peeled and cut in half-slices
½ cup soybeans ***	
Seasoned salt to taste	Seafood seasoning to taste
4 tbs. diet or regular margarine	Juice of 1 lemon
	Dash sea salt ***

Place steaks in a one- or two-inch-deep pan, sprinkle with seasoned salt, sea salt and seafood seasoning. Pour lemon juice over fish. Spread dabs of diet or regular margarine on fish and then cover with soybeans. Put in oven on bake at 325 degrees for 15 minutes. Then turn on broil. After 10 minutes surround fish with apple slices. Broil for 10 more minutes. Place on platter and serve. Serves 4.

*** *Buy in Health Food Store*

SALMON STEAKS WITH MIXED FRUIT

4 medium-sized salmon
    steaks
½ tsp. salt
⅛ tsp. white pepper

Juice of 1 lemon
4 large orange slices
½ cup white seedless grapes
2 tbs. diet margarine

Place steaks in a baking pan. Sprinkle with salt and pepper. Squeeze lemon over all. Dot with diet margarine. Place under broiler for 20 minutes. Cover with orange slices and grapes and bake for 10–15 minutes. Serve with Spinach Ring ** filled with tiny whole beets or buttered carrots. Skip bread that day in order to enjoy beets or carrots. Serves 4.

SAUMON AU TARRAGON

3 lbs. fresh or frozen sal-
    mon, uncooked and cut
    into steaks
3 cups water, or more if
    necessary
2 cups cider vinegar
½ lemon, seeded
1 onion (white)
Sea salt to taste ***

2 bay leaves
4 cloves stuck in lemon
6 peppercorns
Less than ¼ tsp. dill weed
Dash white pepper
Artificial sweetener equal to
    1 tbs. sugar
½ tsp. tarragon
Seafood seasoning to taste

Wash and dry salmon steaks and salt them; sprinkle with seafood seasoning. Set fish on plate. Boil the remaining seasonings slowly in the water and vinegar for 15 to 20 minutes. Add sweetener to taste to liquid and continue cooking for 5 minutes. Then put salmon in pot and bring liquid to a boil again. Continue cooking for 20 minutes. Gently take the salmon out of pot. Remove skin and as many bones as possible. Strain a little of the juice over each fish steak. Put fish in refrigerator on platter to cool. Garnish with watercress or parsley before serving. Serves 6. If you are not using all the fish at one sitting, set the unused part in seasoned liquid in refrigerator.

** *See Recipe Index*
*** *Buy in Health Food Store*

SEAFOOD NEWBURG

1-½ cups diced seafood
    (lobster, shrimp
    crab, scallops, or
    clams)
2 tbs. diet margarine
½ cup light cream or whole
    milk

¾ tbs. gluten flour ***
2 tbs. sherry
2 egg yolks, slightly beaten
½ tsp. salt
Dash cayenne

Melt the margarine in saucepan. Cook the seafood in the Mazola over low heat for 5 minutes. Add the flour, stir in the cream and continue stirring until the sauce barely boils. Stir in the sherry and egg yolks. Cook for 1 minute, taste for seasonings, and correct if necessary. Sprinkle with cayenne. Serves 4.

BROILED BUTTERFLY SHRIMPS

2 lbs. large shrimps
8 tbs. diet margarine
Dash garlic powder
1 tsp. salt

½ tsp. white pepper
½ tsp. paprika
Lemon slices for garnish

Shell and clean shrimps. Leave tails on. Melt margarine in saucepan, add garlic powder, salt and pepper. Place shrimp in broiling pan and brush generously with the margarine. Sprinkle with paprika. Broil under moderate heat for 5 minutes. *Do not overcook.* Serve at once. Garnish with lemon slices. Serves 4–6.

BLACK-EYED SNAPPER

2 medium red snappers,
    split in half
24 large black grapes, pitted
Seasoned salt to taste
Dash seafood seasoning
Pinch black pepper
½ cup white wine

1 teaspoon Poissonade ***
    (composed of thyme,
    basil, sariette, green
    anise and flowers of
    lavender)
Juice of one lemon
Watercress for garnish

Place 4 portions of snapper in shallow pan. Season inside and out with seasoned salt and black pepper. Sprinkle with lemon

*** *Buy in Health Food Store*

juice. Add seafood seasoning, Poissonade and white wine. Place in 350-degree oven for 25 minutes. Turn oven on broil and spread grapes over fish. Broil for 10 minutes or until fish is nicely browned and grapes are soft, but not mushy. Place on platter garnished with watercress. Serves 4.

FILET OF SOLE IN DILL SAUCE

6 good-sized individual slices
   of filet of sole, broiled
   brown and cooled
1 pint sour cream substitute
   or, if allowed, sour
   cream
3 tbs. Mayo 7

1 tsp. chopped dill
1 tsp. chopped onions
Dash salt
1 tsp. lemon juice
Artificial sweetener to taste
Minced parsley

Mix Mayo 7 with sour cream and add all other ingredients. Pour over fish. Sprinkle with minced parsley. Serves 4–6.

FILET OF SOLE MEUNIERE

2 lbs. filet of sole
½ tsp. salt
⅛ tsp. pepper

½ tbs. chopped parsley
2 tbs. diet margarine

Wipe the fish with damp paper towel. Season with salt and pepper. Melt the margarine in nonstick pan. Place fish in pan and cook for five minutes on one side. Turn and cook five minutes longer. Sprinkle with chopped parsley. Serves 4–6.

FRIED FILET OF SOLE HG STYLE

2 lbs. filet of sole
½ cup oat flour
2 eggs, beaten
½ tsp. salt

⅛ tsp. pepper
½ tsp. paprika
½ cup safflower oil

Rinse the fish in cold water. Pat dry on paper towel. Season the beaten eggs with salt and pepper. Dip the fish in egg mixture, roll in oat flour and sprinkle with paprika. Fry in hot safflower oil in nonstick pan until golden brown, approximately 5 minutes on each side. Serves 4–6.

FILET OF SOLE WITH WHITE GRAPES

3 extra-large filets of gray sole
2 tbs. margarine or butter
½ tsp. sea salt ***
Juice of 3 lemons
½ cup white wine
1 tbs. seafood seasoning

Dash paprika
Dash chopped parsley
Dash black pepper
½ lb. white grapes
6 radish rosettes
Lemon wedges for garnish
Parsley bouquets for garnish

Wash fish and dry on paper towel. Set in pan and brush with margarine or butter. Sprinkle with pepper, sea salt or salt substitute, and paprika. Set in lower shelf of oven on broil. Leave for 10 minutes and then add white wine, pouring slowly over fish. Sprinkle with seafood seasoning. Set oven to 350 degrees; leave for another 10 minutes. Remove grapes from vine and place in saucepan. Add enough water to keep from burning. Cook until tender. Place fish on serving platter and sprinkle with chopped parsley. Pour grape mixture over fish. Decorate platter with lemon wedges and bouquets of parsley and rosettes of radishes. Serves 6.

TUNA RING

2 7-oz. cans water-packed tuna
4 eggs (separated)
¾ cup chopped onions

¼ tsp. Italian seasoning
¼ tsp. garlic steak seasoning
½ cup fat-free milk
Pinch of salt

Put tuna, water and milk in blender with onions and egg yolks, seasonings and salt. Blend on Chop and then shift to Whip until smooth. Beat 4 egg whites until stiff. Add pinch of salt. Put tuna in large mixing bowl. Add stiffly beaten egg whites. Then put entire mixture in a 1-½-qt. ring mold that is well greased. (That's the trick in getting it out!) Set mold in shallow pan of water. Bake in a 350-degree oven for 50 minutes, until silver knife inserted in mold comes out clean. Serve with our special Mushroom Sauce.** Serves 6.

** *See Recipe Index*
*** *Buy in Health Food Store*

Vegetables

This Recipe Can Be Used as an Hors d'Oeuvre or Appetizer as Well.

ARTICHOKE BOTTOMS AND CHOPPED VEAL

1 lb. chopped veal
½ cup finely chopped onions
1 egg
4 oz. dry red wine
½ tsp. garlic salt

2 cans artichoke bottoms,
7–10 in can
Chopped parsley

Drain artichokes on paper towel and sprinkle with garlic salt. Combine the veal, onion, egg and wine. Mix well and stuff the artichoke bottoms. Sprinkle the top with freshly chopped parsley. Place under broiler for 8–10 minutes. This mixture will stuff 20 artichoke bottoms.

ARTICHOKE HOLLANDAISE

2 whole artichokes
Dash salt or salt substitute
Dash pepper
Hollandaise Sauce **

Chicken or beef bouillon
cube, depending on main
course

Wash and trim artichokes. Cook in 2 quarts of salted boiling water with chicken or beef cubes until tender—for about 40 minutes. Serve with Hollandaise Sauce or just eat plain. Serves 2.

ARTICHOKES AND MUSHROOMS

4 tbs. butter
2 pkgs. frozen artichokes
½ lb. fresh mushrooms,
sliced

1-½ cups thin cream sauce or
regular milk
3 tbs. sherry

Simmer the artichokes and mushrooms separately in butter or margarine until tender. Combine with Cream Sauce ** and bring to slow boil. Add sherry. Serves 4–6.

* See Recipe Index

104

ARTICHOKE FLOUR SHELLS HG STYLE

½ cup artichoke flour
   shells ***
1 chicken bouillon cube

2 cups boiling water
1 tbs. diet margarine or
   butter

Dissolve the chicken bouillon cubes in boiling water. Add the shells. Cook for 10 minutes. Drain. Add the margarine and toss lightly. Serves 2.

ARTICHOKES IN WHITE WINE

4 to 6 artichokes
Juice of 1 lemon
¼ cup safflower oil
Salt and pepper to taste

4 to 6 minced scallions
½ cup dry white wine
½ clove garlic (minced)
2 tsp. prepared mustard

Wash and trim any coarse outer leaves from medium-sized artichokes. Cover with salted boiling water and cook for 5 minutes, then drain. Stand the artichokes upright on the bottom of a large pot, separate the leaves, pour in the lemon juice, oil, and sprinkle with salt and pepper to taste. Sprinkle with the minced scallions and the ½ cup wine mixed with the garlic and mustard. Cover tightly and simmer large artichokes for 25 to 30 minutes, smaller ones for 20 minutes. If they become dry, add a little oil and wine. Lift them onto individual plates. This is a delicious dish for first course or as a vegetable. Serves 6–12, depending on portions.

ASPARAGUS AND ALMONDS

1 bunch fresh asparagus
Salt and pepper to taste
½ cup melted diet margarine

½ cup evaporated milk
½ cup almonds, toasted and
   ground

Wash and trim the asparagus, tie in a bunch. Stand in boiling salted water and cook until just tender, not mushy. Combine salt, pepper, margarine, milk and nuts and bring to a boil. Place the asparagus on serving dish and pour over the sauce. Serves 4–6.

*** *Buy in Health Food Store*

ASPARAGUS TIPS VINAIGRETTE

24 fresh asparagus tips (canned can be substituted)
1 qt. boiling salted water

Cook the asparagus in boiling salted water until barely tender. Drain and chill. If canned asparagus is used, just drain and chill.

Vinaigrette Dressing

1 tsp. minced onion or ⅛
    tsp. powdered onion
¼ tsp. sugar-free mustard **
⅛ tsp. salt

Dash white pepper
2 tbs. white vinegar
1 tbs. safflower oil

Combine all the ingredients. Chill. Pour over asparagus tips before serving. Serves 4.

Artichoke hearts can be substituted for asparagus tips.

CARROT AND ORANGE RING

8 carrots
½ cup diced onions
Salt and pepper to taste
½ tsp. mace
2 tbs. diet margarine
1 tbs. grated orange rind
½ cup orange juice

Juice of ½ lemon
Artificial sweetener equal to
    2 tbs. sugar
3 egg yolks
2 tbs. gluten flour ***
3 egg whites, beaten

Peel, slice and cook the carrots in a small amount of water, add onion and seasonings. Place in blender and purée with the egg yolks, sweetener, and gluten flour. Gradually add the orange juice. Beat the egg whites until stiff, fold into the purée mixture. Place in a greased 1-½-qt. baking dish and stand in a pan of hot water. Bake in a 350-degree oven for 30 minutes. Serves 6–8.

** *See Recipe Index*
*** *Buy in Health Food Store*

CAULIFLOWER WITH RICE WAFER SAUCE

1 medium-sized cauliflower   1-½ tsp. salt
2 qts. boiling water

Remove the green leaves and rough stem from cauliflower. Cook in boiling salted water until tender, approximately 14 minutes. Drain.

Rice Wafer Sauce

2 rice wafers ***   Dash salt and pepper
2 tbs. diet margarine   Dash paprika

Crush the wafers into crumbs. Sprinkle on top of the cauliflower. Melt the margarine and season with salt and pepper. Pour over the cauliflower. Sprinkle with paprika. Place under the broiler for 5 minutes to brown. Serves 4–6.

EGGPLANT PANCAKES

1 medium eggplant   ½ tsp. salt
2 tbs. sugar-free catsup ***   ⅛ tsp. white pepper
1 tbs. minced onion   1 egg
½ tsp. garlic powder   ½ cup soy flour ***

Peel and grate eggplant. Add egg and beat in. Add seasonings and continue to mix. Sift the flour in slowly. Drop by tablespoon onto a nonstick skillet which has been oiled very lightly. Serves 4.

EGGPLANT PANCAKES WITH DILL

1 eggplant (1 lb.)   ⅛ tsp. garlic powder
2 eggs   ⅛ tsp. dill weed
½ cup gluten flour ***   ½ tsp. paprika
2 tbs. sugar-free catsup ***   1 tsp. parsley flakes
1 tsp. salt   2 tbs. minced onion
⅛ tsp. pepper

*** *Buy in Health Food Store*

Cook eggplant in boiling salted water until just tender. Plunge into cold water. Remove skin and mash pulp. Add the seasonings and mix well. Add the eggs and beat well. Add the flour. Stir until mixture is fairly smooth. Drop by tablespoons into nonstick frying pan. You may use a little safflower oil for frying. Cook until golden brown on both sides. Serves 6–8.

EGGPLANT SOUFFLÉ

1 eggplant weighing 2 lbs.
1 tbs. lemon juice
¼ cup artificial coffee
   creamer

6 egg yolks
6 egg whites
½ tsp. salt
Dash pepper

Cook eggplant unpeeled in salt water until tender. Remove from water. Peel and chop. Place in blender. Add seasonings. Beat egg yolks until light and lemon colored. Add to eggplant. Fold in stiffly beaten egg whites. Lightly grease soufflé dish. Pour mixture into dish. Set into pan of hot water in 450-degree oven for 45–50 minutes, or until a knife inserted into center comes out clean. Serves 4–6.

ENDIVE FROMAGE

2 lbs. Belgian endive
1 qt. boiling water
½ tsp. salt
¼ cup melted diet or regular
   margarine, or butter
½ lb. Parmesan cheese
   (grated)

⅛ tsp. white pepper
½ cup non-dairy coffee
   creamer or evaporated
   milk

Wash the endive. Remove core and cook in boiling salted water until tender. Drain and chill. Grease a 12 × 8-inch baking dish with a little of the butter or margarine. Place layers of endive on bottom of baking dish. Top with cheese and margarine; sprinkle with white pepper. Repeat until ingredients are finished. Top with coffee creamer or milk. Bake in 350-degree oven until brown and bubbly, approximately 35 minutes. Serves 4–6.

PANNED EGGPLANT

1 large eggplant	⅛ tsp. pepper
Soy flour ***	Cottonseed or soy oil ***
½ tsp. salt	

Wash eggplant, cut into ¾ inch crosswise slices. Dry on paper towel. Dip in soy flour seasoned with salt and pepper. Heat small amount soy flour, cottonseed or soy oil in large nonstick pan. Add eggplant. Cook until brown on one side. Turn and brown on the other side. Cooking time: 15–20 minutes. Serves 4.

RED-CAP EGGPLANT

Start Your Charcoal Fire Half an Hour Before Barbecuing This Delicious Dish:

2 large eggplants	Dash Italian seasoning
6 medium-sized tomatoes	1 tsp. diet margarine or
½ tsp. salt	butter
Dash pepper	2 large or 6 small onions
Dash garlic salt	

Peel eggplants. Slice them 1-½ inches to 2 inches thick. Grease lightly with margarine or butter. Add seasonings. Place on top of outdoor grill, covered with silver foil. When slightly tender, top each slice with a slice of white onion about ¼ inch thick, and cap onion with a slice of tomato at least ½ inch thick. Serve when tomatoes, onions, and eggplant are tender. This dish is decorative on meat or fish platters. Serves 6.

MUSHROOMS IN CREAM SAUCE

1 lb. fresh mushrooms, sliced	1 tsp. salt
½ lb. bacon	⅛ tsp. pepper
¼ cup onions, chopped	½ tsp. celery salt
2 tbs. soy flour ***	1-½ cups milk
Juice of half a lemon	3 tbs. sherry

Cook the bacon until crisp. Drain on paper towel. Cool and

*** *Buy in Health Food Store*

109

crumble. Drain half of the drippings from pan. Cook the mushrooms in the remaining drippings until tender. Stir in the flour and seasonings. Add milk and cook over low heat until thickened. Add sherry. Sprinkle with crumbled bacon. Serves 4.

MUSHROOMS AND SOUR CREAM

1 lb. fresh mushrooms, sliced
4 tbs. safflower oil
1 cup onions, chopped
2 tbs. oat flour ***
2 tbs. fat-free milk

1 cup sour cream or sour
   cream substitute
1 tsp. salt
1/8 tsp. white pepper
1/2 tsp. paprika

Sauté the onion in oil until soft. Sprinkle with oat flour, add salt, pepper, and paprika, then stir in milk. Add half of the sour cream. Bring to just below the boiling point, add the mushrooms, cover and simmer for 10 minutes. Mix in the remaining sour cream. Heat thoroughly and serve. Serves 4.

ALMOND-STUFFED ONIONS

4 Spanish onions
1/2 cup chopped toasted
   almonds
1/4 cup Arti Stix,***
   crumbled

1/4 cup diet margarine, melted
1/2 tsp. salt
1/8 tsp. pepper
1-1/2 cups light cream

Peel the onions. Cook in lightly salted water for 10 minutes. Cool. Scoop out the centers. Mix the next 5 ingredients. Stuff the centers of the onions with this mixture. Place in a shallow baking pan. Pour in the cream and bake in a 350-degree oven for 40 minutes. Serves 4.

SAUTÉED PEPPERS

4 sweet green peppers
2 tbs. margarine

1/4 tsp. salt
Dash pepper

Cut the peppers in half. Remove the seeds and white membrane. Chop. Place in skillet with melted margarine, salt and pepper; cook until tender. Serve as a vegetable or hot relish. Serves 2–4.

*** *Buy in Health Food Store*

FRIED POTATOES HG STYLE

4 medium-sized potatoes
2 tbs. minced onions
½ tsp. salt

⅛ tsp. pepper
4 tbs. diet margarine
  (melted)

Peel the potatoes and cut into ⅛-inch thick slices. Brush with melted margarine. Sprinkle with salt and pepper. Fry in a non-stick pan until tender, approximately 20 minutes. Add the onions to pan five minutes before the potatoes are cooked. Serves 4–6.

SPINACH CUSTARD

2 cups cooked spinach,
  chopped
2 tbs. melted margarine
2 eggs, beaten
1 cup milk
¼ tsp. onion juice

⅛ tsp. nutmeg
½ tsp. salt
Dash pepper
Vinegar or lemon juice to
  taste

Mix all the ingredients together. Pour into a buttered casserole. Bake in a 300-degree oven 30 minutes or until firm. Serves 4–6.

Even the Anti-spinach Group Can't Help Enjoying Our Spinach Dishes.

SPINACH DELIGHT

1-½ lbs. spinach, cooked and
  drained
1 small onion

4 slices bacon or kosher fry
  beef
2 tbs. chopped sour pickle

Cut bacon in small slices. Slice onion. Cook bacon and onion over low flame until crisp and onion is yellow. Stir in the pickle and drained cooked spinach. Reheat. Salt if desired. Serves 4.

SPINACH RING I

2 10-oz. pkgs. frozen
    chopped spinach
½ cup fresh mushrooms,
    sautéed
3 eggs, beaten
4 tbs. safflower oil
1 tsp. salt

¼ tsp. white pepper
1 tsp. onion juice
½ cup gluten flour or 1-½
    cups of bread crumbs
    from our bread recipes
¼ cup whole milk or fat-free
    milk

Cook and drain spinach. Place in electric mixer until very fine. Add eggs, cream, oil, salt and pepper and onion juice. Mix in gluten flour or breadcrumbs. Lightly fold in sautéed mushrooms. Pour into a 2-qt. ring mold and bake at 350 degrees for 30 minutes or until firm. Unmold and fill center with tiny boiled white onions and garnish with tiny whole beets or Belgian carrots. Serves 4.

SPINACH RING II

2 10-oz. bags fresh spinach
2 eggs
Salt to taste

2 tbs. diet margarine
2 cups fresh or canned
    mushrooms, sliced

Use 2 plastic bags of spinach. Remove from bags. Chop fine. Sprinkle with salt. Cook over low heat until leaves are tender. Drain. Chop. Season with salt and add diet margarine. Beat 2 eggs until foamy. Fold into spinach mixture. Press into a ring mold spread with margarine. Set mold in hot water. Place in 350-degree oven for 30 minutes. Unmold onto a hot serving plate. Fill center with 2 cups fresh boiled or heated canned mushrooms, sliced. Serves 4.

ACORN SQUASH WITH APPLESAUCE

3 acorn squashes
½ cup organic apple-
    sauce ***
2 tbs. diet margarine

2 tbs. butter
1 tsp. salt
¼ tsp. nutmeg

Cut the squashes into halves and remove seeds. Brush with melted margarine. Sprinkle ½ tsp. salt over. Place cut side down in a shallow pan. Bake in a 350-degree oven for 35 minutes or until

*** *Buy in Health Food Store*

tender, scoop out flesh from shells and squash pulp. Reserve shells. Add applesauce, margarine, nutmeg and salt. Pile the mixture into shells, dot with butter and bake in a 350-degree oven for 25 to 30 minutes. Serves 4–6.

ACORN SQUASH WITH GRAPES

2 medium-sized acorn
  squashes
Artificial sweetener to taste

2 teaspoons diet margarine
32 seedless grapes

Cut squashes in half. Scoop out the seeds. Fill center with diet margarine and artificial sweetener to taste. Bake in 350-degree oven for 30 minutes. Then add 8 seedless grapes to each portion of squash. Set oven on broil for 10 minutes or until grapes are soft, but not mushy. Serves 4.

ACORN SQUASH WITH STRAWBERRIES

2 medium-sized acorn
  squashes
20 strawberries

4 pkgs. artificial sweetener
2 tsp. diet margarine

Cut squashes in half and scoop out seeds. Put margarine in bottom of each squash cup with one package of the artificial sweetener. Bake in 350-degree oven for 30 minutes. Then fill each half with 5 good-sized strawberries. Bake for another 10 minutes and then serve. This squash is particularly good with duck, turkey and Cornish hen. Serves 4.

BAKED ACORN SQUASH

2 medium-sized acorn
  squashes
2 pats of regular or diet
  margarine

4 tsp. powdered artificial
  sweetener
Pinch of salt

Cut squashes in halves and scoop out seeds. Put pat of regular or diet margarine and teaspoon of artificial sweetener and pinch salt in each half. Bake in 375-degree oven for 25–30 minutes until tender. Serves 4.

SQUASH PUDDING

1 yellow squash
6 egg yolks, beaten
6 egg whites, beaten
2 tsp. hot mustard
1 tsp. garlic powder

½ tsp. caraway seeds
Juice of one lemon
1 tsp. salt
⅛ tsp. white pepper
½ cup minced onion

Wash the squash and pat dry on paper towel. Do not peel. Grate, using rough side of the grater. Put in large saucepan. Add the beaten egg yolks, seasonings, lemon juice, and onion. Fold in egg whites. Pour mixture into casserole and bake in 350-degree oven for 45 minutes. Serves 6–8.

STUFFED ACORN SQUASH

2 large acorn squashes
½ cup onion, chopped
⅓ cup safflower oil

1 tsp. salt
⅛ tsp. pepper
2 tbs. heavy cream

Wash the squashes, cut in half and remove seeds. Place in baking pan in a 350-degree oven for 30 minutes, or until tender. Scoop out the pulp. Save the shells. Sauté the onion in oil. Add salt and pepper. Mash the pulp, add the onion, beat in heavy cream. Stuff the shells with mixture and place under broiler until lightly browned. Serves 4.

YELLOW SQUASH PANCAKES

3 cups yellow squash, grated
3 eggs
1 tbs. ketchup or mild sugar-
    free mustard ***
2 tbs. minced onion

1 cup soy flour ***
Safflower oil for frying
Salt and pepper, to taste
Parsley or watercress garnish

Using the coarse side of a grater, grate 3 cups of yellow squash. Add 3 eggs and seasoning. Beat with wire whisk. Gradually add 1 cup of soy flour. Beat until smooth. Heat nonstick frying pan, adding enough oil to cover bottom of pan. Drop pancake batter by tablespoons into hot oil. Fry until golden brown. Turn and brown on the other side. Remove from pan and place

*** *Buy in Health Food Store*

on paper towel to remove any excess oil. Place on warm platter garnished with parsley or watercress. Serve with meat or fish. Serves 6.

STUFFED BAKED TOMATOES

6 large unblemished tomatoes
2 ozs. bacon or kosher fry beef

Wash tomatoes and dry with paper towel. With spoon, scoop out some of the pulp, enough to make room for filling. Set on small pan. Fry bacon or fry beef in nonstick pan until crisp. Place on paper towel to drain fat. Cut up bacon in smallish bits. Spoon bacon bits into openings in tomatoes. Put pan in 350-degree oven. Bake until tomatoes are tender and juicy. *Don't wait until they start wrinkling!* This makes a delicious first course with deviled eggs, or as a side dish for an omelet or steak. Serves 6.

BAKED TURNIPS

1 medium-sized yellow turnip
2 tbs. safflower oil
1 tsp. salt
1/8 tsp. pepper

Artificial sweetener equal to 2 tsps. sugar
1/2 tsp. oat flour ***
2 eggs, separated

Peel the turnip, cut into cubes, wash in cold water. Cook in boiling salted water until tender, about 30 minutes. Drain, mash well. Add other ingredients except eggs. Beat the egg yolks until lemon colored. Gradually stir into the hot mashed turnips. Beat the egg whites until stiff. Fold into the turnip mixture. Pour into a casserole and bake in a 350-degree oven for 30 minutes. Serves 6.

FRIED TURNIPS

1 large white turnip
1 tsp. Italian seasoned salt

Diet margarine
Pinch pepper

Peel turnip and cut into slices, using a French-fry cutter. Brown in nonstick pan with margarine and seasoned salt and pepper. Serves 6.

*** *Buy in Health Food Store*

SPRINGTIME VEGETABLE PLATTER

1 lb. carrots
1 bunch asparagus (1-½ to 2 lbs.)
½ cup Mayo 7
⅓ cup light cream

2 tbs. sour pickle, chopped
1 tbs. black olives, chopped
2 tbs. diet margarine, melted
1 tbs. pimiento, chopped
2 tbs. chopped scallions

Peel and slice the carrots. Trim the asparagus. Cook separately in boiling salted water until tender. Mix together the Mayo 7 and light cream. Cook in a double boiler until the mixture thickens. Stir in the scallions, pickle, olives and pimiento. Keep hot. Drain the asparagus and arrange in a cartwheel shape on a round platter. Top with sauce. Toss the carrots with melted margarine and pile in the center of platter. Serves 6–8.

ZUCCHINI CASSEROLE

2 large zucchini
3 large tomatoes
6 medium-sized white onions
1 tbs. diet margarine or butter

¼ cup Cheddar, crumbled
Dash salt
Dash Italian seasoning
Dash bouquet garni
Dash black pepper

Grease 1-½-quart casserole. Cut up zucchini and tomatoes in large wedges. Peel onions and leave whole. Put zucchini in casserole, add all seasonings, and put in 350-degree oven. After 20–25 minutes or when zucchini begins to grow tender, add tomatoes and onions and bake another 15 minutes. Sprinkle casserole with crumbled Cheddar and bake mixture for another 5–10 minutes. Be sure not to allow the casserole to become mushy. Serves 4–6.

ZUCCHINI PANCAKES

4 cups grated zucchini
2 eggs
3 tbs. minced onion
1½ tsp. salt
⅛ tsp. pepper

½ cup soy flour ***
1 tbs. chopped parsley
½ tsp. paprika
Safflower oil for frying

Wash and grate the unpeeled squash. Use rough side of grater,

*** *Buy in Health Food Store*

116

add the eggs and mix well. Shake in flour and seasonings. Beat with a wire whisk. Cover bottom of skillet with oil. Drop mixture by tbs. into oil. Cook until nice and brown on both sides. Serves 6.

ZUCCHINI PARMESAN

4 cups zucchini, thinly
   sliced
1 small onion, chopped
1 tbs. water
3 tbs. diet margarine

1 tsp. salt
Dash pepper
3 tbs. freshly grated Parmesan cheese

Combine all the ingredients except cheese in skillet. Cover and cook for 2 minutes. Uncover. Turn with a spatula. Cook until barely tender. Place in a serving dish and sprinkle with cheese. Serves 6–8.

STUFFED ZUCCHINI

6 medium-sized zucchini
½ cups Arti Stix crumbs ***
¼ cup minced onion
2 tbs. chopped parsley
1 tsp. salt

⅛ tsp. pepper
2 eggs, beaten
½ cup grated cheese
2 tbs. diet margarine

Wash the zucchini, cut off the ends. Drop into boiling salted water. Cook until barely tender. Cut in half lengthwise. Scoop out the seeds, carefully scoop out the pulp and mash it with a fork, mix in the remaining ingredients except the margarine and cheese. Pile the mixture into the cooked zucchini shells, dot with margarine, sprinkle with cheese. Bake in 350-degree oven for 30 minutes. Serves 6–8.

*** *Buy in Health Food Store*

Casseroles

BROCCOLI AND SHRIMP CASSEROLE

2 pkgs. frozen broccoli
spears
1-½ cups cooked shrimp
2 tbs. diet margarine
2 tbs. gluten flour ***

1-¼ cups milk
1 cup Cheddar, grated
½ tsp. tarragon
Salt and pepper to taste

Cook broccoli according to package directions; drain. Arrange half the broccoli in bottom of a greased 2-qt. casserole and top with cooked shrimp. Sprinkle with salt, pepper and half the tarragon. Add another layer of broccoli. Melt the margarine in a saucepan, blend in flour, salt and pepper to taste and the remaining tarragon. Gradually stir in the milk. Cook until thickened. Stir in ½ cup of Cheddar, stir until cheese melts, pour over the broccoli and shrimp. Sprinkle top with remaining cheddar. Bake in a 350-degree oven for 25 minutes or until cheese is browned. Serves 4–6.

CHICKEN HERB CASSEROLE

1 4–5 lb. roasting chicken
or capon, cut up
2 tbs. bacon fat or kosher
fry beef
Butter or diet margarine
6 tbs. gluten flour ***
3 cups milk
2-½ tbs. salt

Dash pepper
¾ tsp. dried thyme
¾ tsp. dried sage
Dash paprika
Dash chives
Sour cream or sour cream
substitute for garnish
(optional)

Wash, then dry pieces of chicken. Remove excess fat. In heavy skillet cook pieces of chicken in bacon or beef fat (a few at a time) turning until golden. Then place side by side in 2-qt. casserole. Preheat oven to 325 degrees. Add enough butter or margarine to remainder of the fat in skillet to make up 6 ozs. Add flour, blend until smooth, then stir in other ingredients. Cook

*** *Buy in Health Food Store*

until smooth and thickened. Pour sauce over chicken and bake uncovered about 1 hour, or until fork-tender. Garnish with dabs of sour cream or sour cream substitute. Serves 6.

HAM AND NOODLE CASSEROLE

2 cups De Boles Noodles ***
1 cup sour cream
1 cup diced cooked ham
½ cup ripe olives
½ cup chopped soybean
    nuts ***
1 3-oz. can chopped mush-
    rooms (drained)
1 tsp. prepared, sugar-free
    mustard ***
    (Dijon mustard, avail-
    able in grocery stores,
    is suitable.)
⅛ tsp. pepper
1 8-oz. can Cheddar cheese
    soup
1 cup sharp Cheddar, grated

Cook noodles according to package directions. Combine with the other ingredients (except Cheddar). Put in a shallow baking dish, sprinkle with cheese. Bake in a 350-degree oven for 35 minutes, or until bubbly and cheese browns. Serves 6.

MACARONI SHELLS AND CHEESE

1 8-oz. pkg. De Boles
    Shells ***
2-½ qts. boiling water
4 chicken bouillon cubes
1 cup Cheddar, grated
2 cups evaporated milk
2 egg yolks
½ cup Arti Stix,***
    crumbled

Cook the shells in boiling water and bouillon cubes. Place in a 2-qt. baking dish. Combine the next 3 ingredients, pour over the shells and top with Arti Stix crumbs. Bake in a 350-degree oven for 45 minutes. Serves 8–10.

*** *Buy in Health Food Store*

NOODLE AND BEEF CASSEROLE

1-½ lbs. ground beef
1 egg
1 tsp. sugar-free Worcestershire sauce
Dash Tabasco
1 tsp. salt
⅛ tsp. pepper
3 large tomatoes, peeled and diced
1 12-oz. can V-8 juice

¼ tsp. oregano
3 or 4 shakes garlic powder
2 tbs. safflower oil
1 8-oz. pkg. De Boles Noodles
2-½ qts. boiling water
3 tsp. powdered beef broth
1 tsp. salt
Grated Cheddar, if desired

Combine the first 6 ingredients. Mix well and shape into medium-sized meatballs. Place in a nonstick pan and brown on all sides. Remove from pan. Drain off fat. Add the oil and the diced tomatoes to the pan. Cook a few minutes, then add the V-8 juice, oregano and garlic powder. Heat and pour over the meatballs in a 2½-qt. casserole. Cover and bake in 350-degree oven for 30 minutes. Cook the noodles in 2-½ qts. boiling water seasoned with beef broth mix and 1 tsp. salt until just tender. Drain and add to the meat dish. Mix well. Return to the oven and cook until it bubbles, about 20 minutes. Sprinkle with grated Cheddar, if desired. Serves 4–6.

NOODLE MOUSSE

1 8-oz. pkg. De Boles Noodles ***
2-½ qts. boiling water
3 chicken consommé cubes
1-½ cups milk
¼ cup melted diet margarine
2 eggs, beaten

1 pimiento, diced
1 green pepper, diced
1 tbs. onion, chopped
1 tsp. salt
½ cup Cheddar, grated
½ cup crumbled Arti Stix ***

Cook the noodles in boiling water and consommé cubes until tender. Drain and add milk, melted margarine, eggs, pimiento, green pepper, onion, salt, and cheese. Mix well. Place in a greased 2-½-qt. baking dish. Top with crumbled Arti Stix and bake in a 350-degree oven for 40 minutes. Turn out onto a serving platter. Serve with fish or meat. Serves 6–8.

*** *Buy in Health Food Store*

PINEAPPLE, CHICKEN, AND SPAGHETTI CASSEROLE

4 cups cooked chicken,
   cubed
½ lb. mushrooms
4 tbs. diet margarine
2 tbs. soy flour ***
2 cups water or skimmed
   milk

2 chicken bouillon cubes
6 slices dried, sugar-free
   pineapple
½ cup peanuts
Salt and pepper to taste
1 8-oz. pkg. De Boles
   Spaghetti ***

Cook the mushrooms in 2 tbs. margarine until tender. Place in blender and purée for 1 minute. Melt remaining margarine in skillet, add soy flour and blend in; gradually add the 2 cups water or skim milk and chicken bouillon cubes. Cook over low heat until mixture bubbles. Set aside. Cook spaghetti according to package directions. Drain. In a 2-qt. casserole mix the spaghetti, chicken and sauce, add a little salt and pepper to suit your taste. Top with slices of pineapple and sprinkle with peanuts. Bake in a 350-degree oven until heated through, about 45 minutes. Serves 6–8.

PORK CASSEROLE

2 lbs. boneless pork, cut in
   1-inch cubes
¼ cup safflower oil
1 cup chopped onions
1 clove garlic, minced
½ cup chopped green
   pepper
2-½ cups beef bouillon

3 cups sugar-free tomato
   sauce ***
½ cup stuffed olives, cut in
   half
2 cups De Boles spaghetti,
   crumbled ***

Sauté the onions and garlic in oil for 5 minutes. Remove from pan. To the oil in pan add the meat cubes and brown on all sides. Combine the meat, onions, garlic, green pepper, tomato sauce, bouillon and salt in a 2-qt. casserole. Cover and bake in 350-degree oven for 30 minutes. Stir in the crumbled spaghetti and bake until tender. Add the olives and bake 5 minutes longer. Serves 6–8.

*** *Buy in Health Food Store*

TUNA AND CASHEW CASSEROLE

1 7-oz. can tuna
1-½ cups chopped cashew
nuts

¼ lb. sliced mushrooms
¼ cup diced onion
2 tbs. diet margarine

Sauté the mushrooms and onions in margarine for 5 minutes. Flake the fish and add to the mushrooms. Add 1 cup of cashews. Place in a greased 1-½-qt. baking dish. Pour following sauce over it, top with ½ cup crushed cashews and bake in a 350-degree oven for 30 minutes. Serves 4–6.

Sauce

2 tbs. diet margarine
2 tbs. soy flour ***
1-¾ cups milk or light cream

1 tsp. salt
⅛ tsp. white pepper

Melt the margarine, gradually add the soy flour; mix to a smooth paste. Slowly add the milk, stir and cook until bubbly. Add salt and pepper.

VEAL AND CHESTNUT CASSEROLE

2-½ lbs. veal cutlet ¼-inch
thick
½ cup gluten flour ***
2 tsp. paprika
2 tsp. salt
1 tsp. freshly ground
black pepper
2 tbs. diet margarine
1 clove garlic, minced
½ cup water

1 pint sour cream substitute
2 cups boiled chestnuts, cut
into quarters
1 tsp. dried basil
1 tsp. oregano
1 tsp. lemon juice
8 halves dried apricots ***,
cut up
¼ cup Marsala wine
2 tbs. soy powder ***

Put veal between 2 sheets of waxed paper and pound with mallet to flatten. Cut into 2-inch by 1-inch strips. Combine flour, paprika, salt and pepper and dredge veal pieces. Heat margarine and garlic in large skillet, brown veal gently, stirring frequently. Add water, scrape bottom of skillet, add sour cream substitute, lower heat to simmer. Add remaining ingredients, except soy powder. Let come to a boil. Mix soy powder with water and pour into a 1-½-qt. casserole. Sprinkle top with a few additional pieces of apricot. Bake 30 to 45 minutes at 350 degrees, covered. Serves 8.

*** *Buy in Health Food Store*

Sauces, Dressings, Toppings and Garnishes

AVOCADO SALAD DRESSING

1 cup ripe avocado, mashed
2 ozs. safflower or cottonseed oil
1 tbs. vinegar
1 tbs. horseradish

2 ozs. white wine
Artificial sweetener to taste
   (approx. ½ pkg.)
¼ cup onion, minced
Salt and pepper to taste

Blend ingredients in electric blender. Chill for 2 hours. Serve as dressing on mixed green salad, chicken, tuna or salmon salad. Makes 2 cups.

AVOCADO DRESSING

1 ripe avocado
1-½ tbs. lemon juice
1 tsp. prepared Dijon
   mustard

2 tbs. evaporated milk
Dash Tabasco
½ tsp. salt
¼ tsp. paprika

Mash the avocado with a fork. Blend in the other ingredients and beat well. Serve as a salad dressing or as a dip for raw vegetables. Makes 1 cup.

BARBECUE SAUCE

½ cup unsweetened Papaya
   Vita ***
½ cup sugar-free tomato
   catsup ***

1 tsp. hot mustard
1 tbs. charcoal seasoning
¼ cup minced onion

Mix ingredients together. Let stand in refrigerator for 6 hours. Brush on broilers, chops, ribs or fish. Makes 1-½ cups.

*** *Buy in Health Food Store*

BLUE CHEESE SALAD DRESSING

6 ozs. blue cheese
2 tbs. safflower oil

4 tbs. lemon juice
1 cup yogurt

Soften cheese at room temperature and mash with a fork. Blend in oil, beat until smooth, add lemon juice and yogurt. Beat well. Chill. You may use your blender. Makes 2 cups.

BRANDY TOPPING

½ cup margarine
Powdered artificial sweetener
    equal to 1 cup sugar
2 tbs. artificial brandy

2 egg yolks, well-beaten
½ cup plain yogurt
2 egg whites, beaten stiff

Cream margarine. Add sweetener slowly. When all is blended, add brandy. Add beaten egg yolks and yogurt. Pour into top of double boiler and cook over hot water until it thickens. Fold in stiffly beaten egg whites. Serves 6.

CAVIAR SPREAD

1 small jar caviar
2 hard-boiled eggs, riced
1 tbs. grated green onion
1 tbs. chopped parsley
½ tsp. sugar-free
    mustard ***

¼ tbs. sour cream or sour
    cream substitute
½ tsp. salt
Dash pepper
¼ tsp. sugar-free Worcester-
    shire sauce ***

Mix all the ingredients together. Chill for 2 hours. Serve as a spread on triangles of toast made from True HG bread **. Makes 1-½ cups.

SALMON CAVIAR WITH SHALLOTS

4 ozs. salmon caviar
2 shallots, chopped fine
1 tbs. chopped chives
1 tsp. chopped parsley

1 hard boiled egg, chopped
    fine or grated
¼ cup Mayo 7

* See Recipe Index
** Buy in Health Food Store

Combine the caviar, shallots, chives and Mayo 7. Mix in half the chopped egg. Place in the refrigerator to chill. Sprinkle with the remaining chopped egg and parsley. Serve with yellow Squash Pancakes.** Makes 1-¼ cups.

BLACK CHERRY SAUCE

1 lb. fresh black cherries
Artificial sweetener equal to 1 cup of sugar
1 cup water

Wash and pit the cherries. Cook in 1 cup of water until soft. Add the sweetener. Place in electric blender and purée for 1 minute. Chill. Serve as a topping for desserts. Makes approx. 2 cups.

FRESH BING CHERRY AND PORT WINE MOLD

½ lb. fresh cherries
1-½ cups water
Artificial sweetener equal to
   ½ cup sugar

¾ cup port wine for cooking
2 tbs. unflavored gelatin

Cook the cherries in water for 5 minutes. Drain; save the liquid. Pit the cherries. Add the sweetener and wine to the liquid. Soften the gelatin in a little cold water and add to the liquid. Heat until gelatin dissolves. Place the pitted cherries in bottom of 1-½-qt. mold. Pour in liquid. Chill in refrigerator until firm. Serves 8–12.

This is especially good served with chicken. Can be used as a relish.

CRANBERRY CRISP MOLD

1 envelope unflavored
   gelatin
¼ cup cold water
½ cup lemon juice
1 cup boiling water

1 orange, unpeeled
2 cups raw cranberries
Artificial sweetener equal to
   1 cup sugar

Dissolve gelatin in cold water, add lemon juice, boiling water and sweetener. Stir until completely dissolved. Chill until syr-

** *See Recipe Index*

upy. Cut the orange into wedges, remove seeds. Put the orange and cranberries through a food chopper, using the coarse blade. Stir the fruit mixture into the syrupy gelatin. Pour into a 1-qt. mold. Chill until set; unmold onto a platter. Good with turkey or veal.

INSTANT CRANBERRY SAUCE

1 lb. fresh cranberries, washed
½ cup sugar-free black cherry soda

Put cranberries through blender with ½ cup sugar-free black cherry soda and serve. Makes 2-½ cups.

CREAM SAUCE

1-½ tbs. gluten flour ***
1-½ tbs. margarine, diet or
    regular
  ½ tsp. salt

Dash pepper
¾ cup evaporated milk
½ cup water

Melt the margarine in pot. Gradually add the flour. Mix to a paste. Slowly add the milk and water. Cook until it bubbles. Add salt and pepper. Yields 1-½ cups.

CRUMB TOPPING

¼ cup soy or gluten flour ***
Artificial sweetener equal to 2 tbs. sugar
2 tbs. melted diet or regular margarine

Combine the flour and sweetener. Add the melted margarine. Mix into a crumb consistency. Use as desired on baked desserts.

CUSTARD SAUCE

2 egg yolks
Artificial sweetener equal to
¼ cup sugar

½ cup regular or nonfat milk
⅛ tsp. vanilla

*** *Buy in Health Food Store*

Beat egg yolks with milk in top of double boiler. Add vanilla. Add sweetener. Cook until slightly thickened. Serve as a topping on jello or fruit dishes. Makes approx. 1-½ cups.

DILL SAUCE

1 egg beaten until fluffy
1 tsp. salt
Dash white pepper
Artificial sweetener to taste
2 tbs. lemon juice

1 tsp. grated onion
2 tbs. fresh dill, chopped
  fine
1-½ cups sour cream or sour
  cream substitute

Mix all the ingredients together and chill. Serve with meat or fish. Makes 2 cups.

FRUIT SALAD DRESSING

Artificial sweetener equal to
  ½ cup sugar
2 tbs. soy powder
2 eggs, beaten light
1 cup unsweetened pineapple
  juice

Juice of 1 orange
Juice of 1 lemon
1 cup yogurt
6 fresh strawberries
1 tsp. Cherry Heering

Combine sweetener and soy powder, add beaten eggs, juices and liqueur. Cook in double boiler over hot water, stirring constantly until slightly thick. Cool. Makes 2-½ cups.

GRAPE AND WHITE WINE SAUCE

2 cups seedless grapes
1 cup dry white wine

Place grapes and wine in saucepan and simmer until grapes are plump and tender and most of the liquid has evaporated. Use as a sauce for fish or chicken. Makes approx. 2 cups.

GUACAMOLE

2 ripe avocados
1-½ tbs. grated onion
2 tbs. lime juice
½ tsp. sugar-free
    mustard ***

2 tbs. Mayo 7
2 tbs. sugar-free catsup ***
⅛ tsp. pepper
Dash paprika
½ tsp. salt

Mash the avocado pulp with a silver fork. Blend in the remaining ingredients except the paprika. Sprinkle paprika on
top. Chill and serve. Makes 1-½ cups.

HAM DIP

1 cup cooked ground ham,
    lean
3 tbs. Mayo 7
2 tbs. sugar-free chili
    sauce ***

1 tbs. prepared sugar-free
    mustard ***
½ tsp. chili powder
¼ package artificial
    sweetener

Mix all the ingredients well, and chill in refrigerator. Serve as
a dip for Yellow Squash Pancakes **. Makes 2 cups.

HOLLANDAISE SAUCE

½ cup diet margarine,
    melted
4 tbs. lemon juice

½ tsp. salt
4 egg yolks

Put egg yolks in blender with lemon juice and salt. Blend for
1 minute. Gradually pour in hot margarine. The mixture will
thicken gradually. Serve while sauce is hot. Makes 1-½–2 cups.

MOCK HOLLANDAISE SAUCE

¾ cup Mayo 7
⅓ cup fat-free milk
1-½ tbs. lemon juice

1 tsp. grated lemon rind
¼ tsp. salt
Dash pepper

Combine the mayonnaise, milk, salt and pepper in a double
boiler. Cook over simmering water until heated. Stir in the
lemon juice and rind. Makes 1-¼ cups.

*** *Buy in Health Food Store*

MERINGUE

4 egg whites
4 tbs. artificial sweetener
1 tsp. vanilla extract

Beat egg whites until stiff. Add vanilla and sweetener. Spoon over dish of jello or berries. Makes 2 cups.

MUSHROOM SAUCE

½ lb. fresh mushrooms,
    chopped
¼ cup celery, chopped
1 medium-sized onion,
    chopped

2 tbs. diet margarine
1-½ cups skim milk
Seasoned salt and white
    pepper to taste

Combine first five ingredients in pot. Simmer until vegetables are tender. Use a slotted spoon to remove ½ of the vegetables. Place them in blender. Blend until smooth. Return to pot with other vegetables. Season to taste. Makes 2 cups.

OUR HG SALAD DRESSING

3 ozs. vinegar
1 oz. water
4 ozs. cottonseed oil
1 tbs. wine vinegar
½ tsp. paprika
⅛ tsp. garlic powder

½ tsp. dried parsley
1 tsp. herb blend for salads
¼ tsp. Bakon Yeast
2 tsp. Laureleaf Lemon
    Pepper Marinade

Combine ingredients in pint jar. Shake vigorously and place in refrigerator. Keep chilled. Shake vigorously again before pouring over salad. Makes 1-½ cups.

OUR PEPPER POT SALAD DRESSING

2 tbs. Laureleaf Lemon
    Pepper Marinade
1 tsp. herb blend for salads
1 tsp. garlic salt
1 tsp. paprika

2 ozs. wine vinegar
2 tbs. water
4 ozs. safflower oil
Dash Tabasco
Pinch salt

Put the ingredients in blender so that they are well-mixed. Then pour into small bottle or jar. Shake vigorously before using. Makes 1 cup.

FROZEN RASPBERRY TOPPING

1 cup whole milk
½ cup fat-free milk
2 tbs. instant powdered milk, fat-free

1 cup sugar-free raspberry syrup
Artificial sweetener to taste

Mix instant milk with whole and fat-free milk in blender. Add syrup and sweetener to taste and Blend or Frappe. Pour into sauce dish and set in freezer for 1 hour before serving. Makes 2-½ cups.

RASPBERRY-COTTAGE CHEESE TOPPING

3 ozs. cottage cheese
3 ozs. milk (from nonfat dried milk)

1 tbs. raspberry syrup
Artificial sweetener may be added, if desired

Blend all ingredients on Whip or Frappe for at least 5 minutes. Pour into serving dish and let chill. Makes ½ cup.

HG SEAFOOD SAUCE

1 bottle sugar-free chili sauce ***
1 tbs. grated onion
¼ cup lemon juice
2 tbs. horseradish

1 tbs. sugar-free Worcestershire sauce ***
½ tsp. salt
⅛ tsp. Tabasco

Combine all the ingredients, chill and serve. If a milder flavor is desired, stir in 2 tbs. of Mayo 7 or sour cream. Makes 1-½ cups.

*** *Buy in Health Food Store*

SHERRY-MUSHROOM SAUCE

1-½ cups sliced mushrooms   Sherry to taste
  2 tbs. shortening   1-½ tbs. soy powder ***
  ½ tsp. garlic salt   ½ tsp. paprika

Sauté mushrooms and shortening in skillet until barely tender. Add seasonings and sherry to taste. Make a paste of soy powder and cold water and add to mushrooms. Simmer for a few minutes. Serve with fish or chicken. Makes 2 cups.

WATERCRESS PLUS DRESSING

This Dressing Is a Delight over Cold Salmon and Almost Any Other Fish.

2 tbs. finely chopped water-   1 tbs. chervil
     cress   1 tsp. dill
1 tbs. chives, finely chopped   ½ cup Mayo 7
1 tbs. tarragon   1-½ cups plain yogurt

Combine all ingredients in blender. Blend for 3 minutes. Let stand in refrigerator for several hours before using. Makes 2 cups.

MOCK WHIPPED CREAM SAUCE

6 ozs. plain yogurt   Artificial sweetener to taste
1 oz. cottage cheese   2 drops red food coloring

Mix all ingredients on Frappe in blender for at least 5 minutes or until mixture is smooth. Makes approx. 1 cup.

YOGURT MIX SAUCE

1 6-oz. container of plain yogurt
2 slices dietetic pineapple
1 tbs. of juice from the pineapple can

Place the pineapple and juice in blender for 30 seconds. Mix in yogurt. Chill. Makes approximately 1-½ cups.

*** *Buy in Health Food Store*

Desserts

FOR THE CLIMAX OF YOUR MEAL:

These Desserts Are Delicious. They Really Satisfy a Craving for Sweets That Has a Nasty Way of Cropping up Now and Again.

You Don't Have to Give up Delicious Desserts—Even Your Favorites—Just Because of Hypoglycemia. For Instance:

APPLE BROWN BETTY HG

10 brown rice wafers ***
¾ container (6-oz.) diet margarine
3 tbs. powdered artificial sweetener

6 ozs. raisins or cranberries (optional—for flavoring)
3 lbs. green apples

Melt margarine. Brush bottom of Pyrex or any suitable oven-to-table bowl with melted margarine. Line bowl with crushed rice wafers. Add a good layer of sliced apples and margarine. Sprinkle raisins on apples. Add 1 tbs. artificial sweetener. Add another layer of crushed wafers, then apples, margarine, raisins or cranberries, artificial sweetener. Then top the ingredients with the crushed wafers and artificial sweetener. Serves 6 to 8, depending on appetites.

APRICOT OR DATE COFFEECAKE

1 cup oat flour ***
¼ tsp. salt
2 tbs. artificial sweetener
2 tsp. baking powder
1-½ tbs. shortening
2 eggs, beaten

3 tbs. cold water
1 tbs. chopped dates * or apricots *
Cinnamon
1 package artificial sweetener

After sifting flour, combine the dry ingredients and work in shortening. Add beaten eggs and water and stir gently. Add

* If dates and apricots are not on your diet use strawberries (raw) or dried unsweetened prunes.
*** Buy in Health Food Store

132

fruit. Spread dough on small greased pie pan, Pyrex or tin. Sprinkle package of artificial sweetener and cinnamon over mixture. Bake in a preheated oven at 425 degrees if gas stove, or 350 degrees in electric stove at least 20 minutes. Serves 4–6.

APRICOT DELIGHT CAKE

1 cup Jolly Joan Oat
   Mix ***
2 cups gluten flour ***
3 cups milk
4 tbs. baking powder
¼ cup safflower oil

Artificial sweetener equal to
   1-½ cups sugar.
1 cup dried apricots, cut up
   fine
½ cup pecans, cut up

Beat oil and sweetener in large mixing bowl. Add milk and flour with baking powder, gradually. Then put in electric mixer for at least 5 minutes or until smooth, slowly tossing in apricots and nuts. Pour into an aluminum or Pyrex loaf pan 9 x 5 x 2-¾ inches. For those who are concerned about their weight, reduce the amount of nuts and apricots. Serves 4–6.

HG APRICOT SOUFFLÉ

1 lb. dried apricots
½ cup cream, whole milk
   or non-dairy coffee
   creamer
Artificial sweetener to taste
8 egg yolks, beaten

¼ cup ground browned
   almonds
1 tsp. almond extract
8 egg whites, beaten
¼ cup sherry

Stew dried apricots in artificial sweetener until soft. Place in blender on Chop for 2 minutes. Add the cream and pour it over the thickly beaten egg yolks. Mix in the fruit, nuts, almond extract and sherry. Beat the 8 egg whites until stiff and mix ¼ of them into the purée mixture, then lightly fold in the rest. Bake for about 60 minutes at 450 degrees in a greased 2-qt. soufflé dish. Serves 4–6.

*** *Buy in Health Food Store*

BLACKBERRY GRAND MARNIER

2 envelopes unflavored
    gelatin
½ cup cold water
Artificial sweetener equal to
    1-¼ cups sugar
Juice of one lime
Pinch cream of tartar

2 pints crushed blackberries
2 egg whites
Pinch salt
4 tbs. Grand Marnier
Yogurt or whipped cream,
    sweetened with artificial
    sweetener

Soften gelatin in cold water in saucepan. Add lime juice and sweetener equal to 1 cup sugar. Stir over low heat until gelatin is completely dissolved. Add crushed berries. Place in refrigerator until mixture starts to thicken. Beat egg whites and add pinch cream of tartar, pinch salt, and artificial sweetener equal to ¼ cup of sugar. Beat on slower speed until white peaks form. Fold in the stiffly beaten egg whites into mixture. Add Grand Marnier. Pour into serving dish. Chill for 4 hours. Top with yogurt or whipped cream, sweetened with artificial sweetener. Serves 4.

BLACKBERRY ICE

3 1-pint boxes blackberries
2 cups cold water
Artificial sweetener equal
    to 1-½ cups sugar

3 envelopes unflavored
    gelatin
Dash salt or salt substitute
Lemon juice to taste

Stew blackberries in 1 cup cold water with artificial sweetener until mushy. Pour through a coarse sieve, ricer or food mill. Dissolve gelatin in ½ cup cold water. Stir over low heat. Add lemon juice to taste, artificial sweetener and salt. Mix well. Pour into 2 refrigerator ice trays and freeze. Makes 1-½ qts. You can follow this recipe for strawberries and raspberries, substituting lime juice for lemon juice. Serve with Frozen Raspberry Topping.** Serves 6–8.

** *See Recipe Index*

BLACKBERRY SPONGE

1-½ envelopes unflavored
    gelatin
2-½ tbs. cold water
Artificial sweetener equal to
    ½ cup sugar
Juice of 1-½ limes
  2 egg whites

1-¼ pints crushed
    blackberries
Yogurt sweetened with
    sugar substitute or
    sugar-free whipped
    cream, for topping.

Soften gelatin in cold water. Add lime juice and sweetener. Stir over low heat until gelatin is completely dissolved. Add crushed berries. Place in refrigerator until mixture starts to thicken. Beat eggs until they form white peaks. Fold the stiffly beaten egg whites into mixture. Chill for 4 hours. Top with yogurt which has been sweetened with sugar substitute or whipped cream. Serves 4.

BLACKBERRY SUPREME

2 cups soy flour
2 eggs
2 cups whole milk or
    non-dairy milk
2 tsp. baking powder
1 stick diet margarine

2 cups blackberries
Artificial sweetener equal to
    1-½ cups sugar
1 tsp. vanilla extract
Cinnamon

In a large mixing bowl, cream margarine and half of the sweetener. Add the eggs and beat. Add the flour and milk and baking powder and mix well with a wire whisk. The batter should be thin enough to pour. Pour into a greased baking dish. Cover with the berries which have been sweetened with remaining sweetener and vanilla. Top with Crumb Topping.** Sprinkle with cinnamon. Bake in 350-degree oven for 50 minutes to 1 hour. Serves 4–6. This dessert will be just as delicious with blueberries.

** *See Recipe Index*

BLUEBERRY OR BLACKBERRY MOUSSE

2 pints blueberries or
blackberries
5 egg yolks, beaten
Artificial sweetener equal to
1 cup of sugar

2 envelopes unflavored
gelatin
½ cup cold water
5 egg whites beaten stiff

Place berries and sweetener in top part of double boiler. Cook until tender. Soften gelatin in cold water and stir until dissolved. Add the beaten egg yolks. Stir until mixture coats a spoon. Fold in the stiffly beaten egg whites. Pour mixture into serving dish and chill for 4 hours. Serves 6.

BLUEBERRY OR RASPBERRY OAT COOKIES

1 egg
Artificial sweetener equal to
½ cup sugar
¼ tsp. vanilla
Pinch salt
1 cup oat flour ***
2 tbs. berries

½ cup melted butter or
margarine
1 tbs. roasted soybeans,
chopped ***
Additional artificial
sweetener for berries

Wash and dry berries, sprinkle lightly with artificial sweetener and let set 5 minutes. Beat egg until smooth and add artificial sweetener gradually. Add remaining ingredients. Preheat oven. Lightly spread butter or margarine on a 14 × 18-inch baking sheet. Form little balls of mixture and set on cookie sheet, over an inch apart. Press down with tines of fork. Bake until brown in a 350-degree oven. After 5 minutes or after cookies have browned lightly, turn cookies upside-down with blade spatula. When cookies are crisp place on platter. Makes 18–24 cookies.

Variations: Strawberry Oat Cookies—substitute 2 tbs. strawberries and 1 tbs. chopped peanuts for the berries and roasted soybeans. Apricot-Oat Cookies—substitute 2 tbs. chopped dried apricots and 1 tbs. chopped almonds for the berries and roasted soybeans.

*** *Buy in Health Food Store*

BLUEBERRY PUDDING

2 pints blueberries
3 egg yolks, beaten
Artificial sweetener equal to
   1 cup of sugar

2 envelopes unflavored
   gelatin
½ cup cold water
5 egg whites, beaten stiff

Place berries and sweetener with water in top part of double boiler. Cook until tender. Add the beaten egg yolks. Stir until mixture coats a spoon. Soften gelatin in cold water, add and stir until dissolved. Cook, when the mixture starts to thicken. Fold in the stiffly beaten egg whites. Pour into serving dishes and chill for 4 hours. Serves 10–12.

BLUEBERRY SNOWBALL

4 tbs. cold water
2 envelopes unflavored
   gelatin
2 cups blueberries

2 cups water
4 tbs. artificial sweetener
1 tbs. Benedictine

Stew berries in water, add sweetener and Benedictine. Soften gelatin in cold water, add to berries. Pour into large dish and chill. Top with Meringue ** before serving. Serves 4–6.

MOCK BLUEBERRY WHIP

4 ozs. yogurt
½ tsp. vanilla
  2 tbs. fresh blueberry juice

Artificial sweetener to taste
1 oz. cottage cheese

Put ingredients into blender and whip for 2 or 3 minutes. Then shift to Frappé for 5 minutes. Pour sauce into serving bowl. Serves 4–6.

MIDNIGHT PUDDING

2 cups fresh blueberries
2 cups blueberry juice and
   water

2 envelopes unflavored
   gelatin
Artificial sweetener to taste

Stew berries for 3 minutes. Soften gelatin in a little cold water. Add to the blueberry juice, add berries, sweeten to taste. Pour into a mold to set, or use individual dishes. Top with mock whipped cream sauce **. Serves 4.

** *See Recipe Index*

CAROB MOUSSE

(Tastes Like Chocolate. Looks Like Chocolate.)

4 tbs. Carob Powder ***
6 egg yolks
1 cup milk

Artificial sweetener to taste
Dash vanilla

Mix 6 egg yolks with sweetener in double boiler. Gradually add milk. Cook until it begins to thicken. Gradually add carob powder and vanilla. Beat with wire whisk and pour into individual dishes. Refrigerate until serving. Serves 4.

CHEESECAKE

2-½ cups cottage cheese
Juice of one lime
2 tsp. walnut extract
3 tbs. safflower oil
5 eggs

1 cup of strawberries,
blueberries or
raspberries
Artificial sweetener equal to
¼ cup sugar

Place the eggs, juice, oil, walnut extract in blender and blend for 1 minute. Slowly add the cottage cheese. Blend until smooth. Pour into 12 x 12-inch cake pan. Sweeten the berries and spread on top. The mixture is thin, so the berries will sink to the bottom. Bake in a 350-degree oven for 1 hour, or until the cake is firm. Turn off the oven and leave the door open. Let the cake cool in the oven. Chilling improves the flavor. Serves 4–6.

HG CHOCOLATE CHEESECAKE

2 cups cottage cheese
4 ozs. yogurt
3 tbs. safflower oil
5 eggs
1 cup gluten flour ***

2 tbs. baking powder
6 tbs. carob powder ***
Artificial sweetener equal to
½ cup sugar, or to suit
your taste

Sift the flour, baking powder, carob powder and sweetener together. Place the eggs and safflower oil in blender. Blend on low speed for 1 minute. Add the cheese and yogurt. Blend on high speed until smooth. Combine mixture with the flour mix-

*** *Buy in Health Food Store*

ture and stir until smooth. Pour into a greased 12 × 12-inch cake pan. Bake in a 350-degree oven for 1 hour. Turn off oven; open the door. Allow cake to remain in oven until cooled. Chill and serve. Serves 6–8.

CREPES SUZETTE HG STYLE

2 eggs
2 tbs. club soda
⅛ tsp. salt

Dash of pepper
½ tbs. diet margarine
Sugar-free strawberry jelly

Beat the egg and soda with a wire whisk; add salt and pepper. Melt the margarine. Drop the egg mixture by tablespoonfuls into pan. Cook until barely firm. Turn and cook for a few more seconds. Place on hot platter, making layers of crepes and jelly. Serves 2.

GELATIN CHEESE TORTE PIE FILLING

1 envelope saccharin-
    sweetened gelatin
1 cup boiling water
8 oz. cream cheese

1-½ tsp. artificial liquid
    sweetener
1-⅓ cups whipping cream

Dissolve gelatin in boiling water. Cool until consistency of raw egg white. Cream together cheese and liquid sweetener. Add gelatin and mix well; whip whipping cream; fold together. Pour filling into crust. Chill several hours or overnight. Serves 4–6.

BING BANG JELLO

2 cups fresh cherries
2 cups cherry juice and
    water

2 envelopes unflavored
    gelatin
Artificial sweetener to taste

Stew cherries for 2 minutes. Drain; reserve liquid. Pit the cherries, soften gelatin in a little cold water; add to the liquid, add the cherries, sweeten to taste. Pour into a mold to set or individual dishes. Serve with Mock Cream Sauce **. Serves 4–6.

** *See Recipe Index*

SUGARLESS CHIFFON CAKE

¾ cup gluten flour
⅓ cup soy flour
1-½ tsp. baking powder
½ tsp. salt
2 tbs. corn oil
4 beaten egg yolks
½ cup cold water

1-½ tbs. lemon juice
1 tsp. lemon rind
1 tsp. vanilla
4 beaten egg whites
¾ tsp. cream of tartar
2 tsp. artificial liquid
    sweetener

Sift flour, baking powder, and salt into small mixing bowl. Make well in center. Add oil, egg yolks, water and lemon juice, rind and vanilla. Beat until smooth. Be careful not to overmix. Beat egg whites until foamy, add cream of tartar, and liquid sweetener. Beat at high speed until very stiff peaks form. Fold in batter until even in color. (Do not stir.) Pour into an ungreased 8-inch or 9-inch square cake pan or a loaf pan. Bake at 300 degrees until top springs back. Invert pan until cool, then remove from pan. For 10-inch tube pan, double recipe. Serves 10.

Printed with permission of Chicago Dietetic Supply, Inc.

CHOCOLATE BAVARIAN

1 tbs. unflavored gelatin
2 tbs. water
1 oz. baking chocolate
    (bitter) *
1 cup whole milk

1 tsp. artificial liquid
    sweetener
½ tsp. vanilla
2 cups whipping cream

Soften gelatin in water. Melt chocolate in milk over boiling water. Add softened gelatin and liquid sweetener, stirring until gelatin dissolves. Remove from heat, add vanilla, and let stand until mixture thickens (consistency of raw egg white). Whip until fluffy on high speed of mixer. In separate bowl, whip cream. Fold together. Spoon into a 4-cup mold. Chill until firm, about 3 hours. Serves 8.

Printed with permission of Chicago Dietetic Supply, Inc.

* For those forbidden chocolates, carob, bought in health food stores, can be substituted.

CINNAMON COOKIES

⅓ cup diet margarine
1 cup gluten flour ***
½ tsp. baking powder
1 tsp. cinnamon
Dash salt

¾ tsps. artificial liquid
    sweetener
1 tsp. vanilla
¼ cup water

Cream margarine, blend in flour, baking powder, cinnamon and salt. Mix vanilla, water and liquid sweetener. Stir into flour mixture and mix thoroughly. Shape dough into 30 balls and flatten with a fork. Bake at 375 degrees for 15 minutes.

Printed with permission of Chicago Dietetic Supply, Inc.

COCONUT PUFFS

1 tsp. artificial liquid
    sweetener ***
1 tsp. gluten flour ***
1 egg white

⅔ cup shredded coconut,
    dry
½ tsp. vanilla

Beat egg white until fluffy, gradually adding liquid sweetener, gluten flour and vanilla. When egg whites stand in peaks, fold in coconut. Drop on greased cookie sheet. Bake at 350 degrees until golden brown. Makes 10 cookies.

Printed with permission of Chicago Dietetic Supply, Inc.

DECAFFEINATED COFFEE-MAPLE JELLO

1-½ envelopes unflavored
    gelatin
2 tbs. cold water
Artificial sweetener equal to
    ½ cup sugar (less or
    more as desired)

2 cups strong hot
    decaffeinated coffee
½ cup artificially sweetened,
    imitation maple
    syrup ***

Soften gelatin in 2 tbs. cold water in saucepan. Add artificial sweetener. Stir over heat until gelatin dissolves. Remove from stove to add coffee and maple syrup. Stir well and then pour into individual dishes or a mold. Chill for 3–4 hours. Serve with

*** *Buy in Health Food Store*

either Mock Whipped Cream Sauce ** or Brandy Topping ** or sugar-free whipped cream. Serves 4.

DECAFFEINATED COFFEE JELLO

2 cups strong hot
   decaffeinated coffee
2 envelopes unflavored
   gelatin
Artificial sweetener equal to
   ½ cup sugar (more or
   less as desired)

¼ cup cold water
½ cup artificial maple
   syrup ***
Yogurt (artificially
   sweetened) or whipped
   cream

Dissolve gelatin in ¼ cup cold water in saucepan. Add sweetener and vanilla and maple syrup. Stir over heat until gelatin dissolves. Remove from stove and add coffee. Stir well, and then pour into individual glass compote dishes or mold. Chill for 3–4 hours. Serve with artificially sweetened yogurt or whipped cream. Serves 4.

CRANBERRY CRUMBLE

Artificial sweetener equal to
   1-¼ cups sugar
2 cups fresh cranberries
1 tbs. orange rind, grated
⅔ cup prunes, cooked and
   chopped

1 cup water
¼ cup oat flour ***
¼ cup butter or diet
   margarine
1 cup Arti-Stix,
   crushed ***

Combine sweetener equal to one cup sugar and water in saucepan. Bring to a boil; add cranberries and continue cooking for 5 minutes or until cranberries burst. Add orange rind and prunes. Pour into a 1-½-qt. casserole. Combine oat flour and remaining artificial sweetener and work in butter or margarine with fork until crumbly; add crushed Arti-Stix and toss. Sprinkle over fruit mixture. Bake at 400 degrees for 45 minutes. Serves 4–6.

** *See Recipe Index*
*** *Buy in Health Food Store*

CRANBERRY SHERBET

1 qt. stewed fresh
   cranberries
Juice of 2 oranges
Juice of 1 lemon

Artificial sweetener equal to
   1 lb. sugar
2 beaten egg whites

Prepare a cranberry sauce made by pressing 1 qt. stewed fresh cranberries through a sieve. Add the sweetener, juice of oranges and lemon. Freeze to a mush. Mix in the beaten egg whites and finish freezing. Can be served with fowl. Serves 4–6.

CREMA DI BAGNOMARIA HG STYLE

2 whole eggs
4 egg yolks
1 cup skimmed milk
Dash nutmeg

Artificial sweetener equal to
   3 tbs. sugar
½ tsp. vanilla

Place the eggs in a large bowl. Add the sweetener and beat well. Gradually add the milk and vanilla. Continue to beat until well mixed. Strain through a fine sieve. Pour into a greased 1-qt. casserole. Place in a pan of hot water. Cook on top of the stove until thickened, at least 1 hour. Do not allow the water in the pan to boil, as it will cause the cream to curdle. Sprinkle with nutmeg and serve hot or cold. Serves 4.

BAKED CUSTARD

1 cup scalded milk (whole
   or skim)
1 beaten egg
½ tsp. artificial liquid
   sweetener

½ tsp. vanilla
⅛ tsp. cinnamon
Dash salt
Pan of water

Add scalded milk slowly to beaten egg. Add the rest of ingredients. Pour into custard cups and place custard cups in pan of water. Bake in 350-degree oven until a silver knife when inserted comes out clean. Serves 2.

Printed with permission of Chicago Dietetic Supply, Inc.

CARIBBEAN CUSTARD

Diet margarine or butter
Artificial sweetener equal to
　　1-½ cups sugar (less, if
　　desired)
1 tsp. almond extract
6 tsp. rum extract
　　(imitation)
1 tsp. vanilla extract

4 eggs
3 cups scalded milk
　　(2 whole milk, 1
　　fat-free)
1-½ tbs. cold water
¼ cup roasted almonds
　　or pistachio nuts,
　　chopped

Grease bottom of 1-qt. casserole dish with margarine or butter. Heat artificial sweetener (amount equal to 1 cup of sugar) with 1-½ tbs. of cold water and stir until powder is entirely dissolved. This is tricky. Be patient. Add rum extract and stir well into a syrup. Pour into bottom of casserole. Put dish into refrigerator for syrup to chill and harden—at least half an hour. Beat eggs lightly using wire whisk, with remaining artificial sweetener, salt, vanilla and almond extract. Add scalded milk gradually and pour mixture into casserole. Set dish in pan with at least 1 inch of water and place in 350-degree oven for 40–45 minutes, or until a silver knife inserted in custard comes out clean. Before the custard is firm sprinkle with roasted almonds or pistachio nuts. Serves 4–6.

FLAN (CARAMEL CUSTARD) HG STYLE

4 eggs
Artificial sweetener equal to
　　1-½ cups sugar (less or
　　more as desired
6 tsp. imitation caramel
　　flavor

Dash salt
3 cups milk, scalded (2
　　whole, 1 fat-free)
1 tsp. vanilla extract
1 tsp. almond extract
1-½ tbs. cold water

Grease bottom of Pyrex bowl or 6 custard cups with margarine or butter. Heat artificial sweetener equal to 1 cup sugar with 1 tbs. cold water and stir until entirely dissolved. (See instructions for Maple Custard HG Style **.) Add syrup and stir until smooth. Pour into bottom of bowl. Set bowl in refrigerator for syrup to cool and harden. Beat eggs lightly using wire whisk, with artificial sweetener equal to ½ cup sugar, salt, vanilla and almond extract. Add scalded milk gradually and pour into bowl. Set bowl in pan with at least 1 inch water and place in 350-degree oven for 40–50 minutes, or until a silver knife inserted in custard comes out clean. Serves 4. Serve with Strawberry Frou Frou **.

FRUIT CREAM QUICKIE

4 nectarines, peeled and
   sliced
3 peaches, peeled and sliced
2 cups yogurt

Artificial sweetener to taste
4 ozs. artificially sweetened
   raspberry syrup

Fill a wide, shallow serving bowl with fruit. Cover the fruit thickly with yogurt which has been sweetened with artificial sweetener equal to 1 cup sugar. Pour raspberry syrup slowly over yogurt and chill. Serves 4.

FRUIT RING

2 envelopes unflavored
   gelatin
¼ cup cold water
¼ cup lime juice
½ cup boiling water
1 cup sugar-free ginger ale
1 8-oz. can dietetic pears,
   drained

1 8-oz. can dietetic pineapple chunks, drained
½ cup seedless grapes
½ cup creamed cottage
   cheese
¼ cup almonds, blanched
   and slivered

Sprinkle the gelatin onto cold water to soften. Add boiling water and stir until dissolved. Add lime juice and ginger ale. Pour ⅓ of the gelatin into mold and place in refrigerator to set. Arrange pears rounded side down on top of the set gelatin. Spoon half of the remaining gelatin around and over the pears. Place in refrigerator again to set. Mix the remaining gelatin with pineapple, grapes, almonds. Fold in the cottage cheese. Pile on top of the chilled gelatin. Chill until set. Unmold onto serving platter. Serves 6–8.

** *See Recipe Index*

BROILED GRAPEFRUIT

Cut grapefruit in half. Loosen sections. Sprinkle with artificial sweetener to taste. Place under broiler for 5 to 7 minutes and serve.

LEMON PUDDING

4 lemons, juice and rind
Artificial sweetener equal to
   1 cup sugar
7 egg yolks, beaten
1 tbs. unflavored gelatin
½ cup cold water
7 egg whites, stiffly beaten
Artificial sweetener equal to
   ¾ cup sugar

¼ cup white crème de
   menthe (arti-
   ficial) ***
1 cup strawberries
1 cup peaches
1-½ packages dietetic
   ladyfingers

Place lemon juice and grated rind and sweetener equal to 1 cup sugar in top of double boiler. Stir until dissolved. Add beaten egg yolks, cook and stir until the mixture coats a silver spoon. Soften gelatin in cold water and add to egg yolk mixture. Stir until dissolved. Remove from heat and cool. Beat egg whites and add sweetener. Fold egg whites into gelatin mixture. Line a spring-form mold with ladyfingers and pour mixture into it. Set in refrigerator for 45 minutes. Slice strawberries and peaches. Stew until barely tender, add crème de menthe when the mixture starts to thicken slightly. Sprinkle the fruit on top. It will gradually sink. Chill for 6 hours or longer. Top with fresh sliced strawberries or peaches and serve. Serves 8–10.

KEY LIME CHIFFON JELLO

1 envelope unflavored
   gelatin
¼ cup cold water
4 eggs, separated
Artificial sweetener equal to
   ½ cup sugar

½ cup lime juice
1 tbs. lemon juice
Grated rind of ½ lime
Green food coloring
Dash salt

Soften gelatin in cold water. Place yolks in top of double boiler. Beat into them salt, ½ of the sweetener, juices, and lime rind. Cook over hot, not boiling, water until mixture coats a spoon.

Remove from stove and add gelatin. Cool until it starts to thicken. Pour into blender. Add green coloring. Blend until light and fluffy. Beat egg whites until stiff. Continuing to beat, add remaining sweetener, 1 tablespoon at a time. Fold into gelatin mixture and pour into mold or deep Pyrex casserole dish. Refrigerate for several hours before serving. Top with Meringue **. Serves 6.

MAPLE CUSTARD HG STYLE

4 eggs
Artificial sweetener equal to
   1-½ cups sugar (less
   or more as desired)
½ cup artificially flavored
   maple syrup ***
Dash salt or salt substitute

3 cups milk, scalded (2
   whole, 1 fat-free)
1 tsp. vanilla extract
1 tsp. almond extract
2 tbs. cold water
1 cup dry roasted peanuts,
   chopped

Grease bottom of 1-qt. Pyrex bowl or 6 custard cups with margarine. Beat artificial sweetener with 2 tbs. cold water and stir until entirely dissolved. This is tricky. Be patient. Add syrup and stir well. Pour into bottom of bowl. Set bowl in refrigerator for syrup to cool and harden. Beat eggs lightly, using wire whisk, with artificial sweetener equal to ½ cup sugar, salt, vanilla and almond extract. Add scalded milk gradually and pour into bowl. Set bowl in pan with at least 1 inch of water and place in 350-degree oven for 45 minutes, or until a silver knife inserted in custard comes out clean. Just before testing (after about 40 minutes) sprinkle custard with chopped dry roasted peanuts. Serves 6.

MAPLE DELIGHT

1 pkg. low-calorie vanilla
   pudding mix
½ cup artificial maple
   syrup ***

1-½ cups milk
artificial sweetener to taste

Empty pudding mix into saucepan. Gradually stir in milk, syrup and sweetener. Stir over heat until mixture comes to a boil. Remove from stove and pour into individual dishes or mold. Let mixture cool before refrigerating. Serves 4.

** See Recipe Index
*** Buy in Health Food Store

FRUIT-STUFFED CRANSHAW MELON

1 Cranshaw melon
2 cups strawberries
2 cups blueberries

1 cup blackberries
4 ozs. raspberry brandy

Cut melon in half. Remove seeds. Scoop out melon balls using large end of baller scoop. Mix melon balls with strawberries, blueberries and blackberries; sprinkle with raspberry brandy. Fill the shell with the fruit and serve. Serves 8.

MELON BALLS CRÈME DE MENTHE

1 cantaloupe
1 honeydew melon
½ watermelon
½ cup white crème de
    menthe (artificial) ***

2 cups fresh blackberries,
    raspberries or
    blueberries
Rhubarb leaves or other
    green leaves for bed

Make enough melon balls so that each person may have the equivalent of 1 cup. Place 2 large rhubarb leaves or the like on bottom of deep compote dish. Fill with assorted melon balls topped with berries. Sprinkle with white crème de menthe. Place in refrigerator 3 hours before serving. Serves 6–8.

BAKED PEACHES OR NECTARINES

This Is a Good Way of Taking Care of an Oversupply of Fruit.

6 peaches or nectarines
6 pkgs. artificial sweetener
1 cup water

½ cup artificially-sweetened
    raspberry syrup

Remove skin from top of fruit. Set in shallow baking pan, sprinkle with sweetener and glaze with the syrup. Pour cup of water in pan and bake in 350-degree oven about 15 minutes, or until peaches are tender. Serves 6.

*** *Buy in Health Food Store*

PEACH BURGUNDY

6 large, fresh peaches
Artificial sweetener equal to 6 tbs. sugar
½ cup Burgundy

Cut the peaches in half, remove pits, and place in baking dish. Sprinkle with sweetener. Pour a little wine into each cavity. Bake in 350-degree oven for 25 minutes. Serves 6.

PEACH CAKE

2 cups soy flour ***
2 tbs. baking powder
2 eggs
2 cups whole milk
8–10 large peaches, sliced

¼ lb. diet margarine or butter
Artificial sweetener equal to 1-½ cups sugar

In a large bowl cream butter and half of the sweetener. Add the eggs. Beat with a wire whisk until smooth. Pour in milk. Sift the flour and baking powder together. Add to the egg mixture. Beat well with a wire whisk. Pour the batter into an 8-inch spring-form pan. Sprinkle the peaches with the other half of sweetener and 2 tablespoons soy flour. Place peaches on top of batter and press down. Bake in 350-degree oven for 1 hour, or until crust is crisp and brown. Serves 6–8.

PEACH MUMBO-JUMBO

1 pkg. low-calorie vanilla pudding mix
1 8-oz. can dietetic peaches

½ tsp. vanilla
1 cup fat-free or whole milk

Empty pudding mix into saucepan. Gradually stir in 1 cup of peach juice from the can and 1 cup of milk. Stir over medium heat until mixture comes to a boil. Allow mixture to cool. Then pour into blender with the peaches and vanilla. Set blender on Whip for about 10 minutes. Pour the contents of the blender into individual dishes and let chill. Serves 4.

*** *Buy in Health Food Store*

LOW-CALORIE PEAR CREAM DELIGHT

½ cup cold water
3 tbs. unflavored gelatin
1 16-oz. can dietetic pears
　plus the juice
3 whole eggs (large)
Berries or melon for garnish

1 cup skimmed milk or
　whole milk
Artificial sweetener to taste
Dash artificial vanilla
½ cup white wine

Place pears and the juice from can in blender. Whirl until smooth. Add the eggs and sweetener. Mix until smooth. Soften gelatin in water. Mix in milk, and heat until gelatin is dissolved. Add to mixture in blender and artificial vanilla. Mix well. Pour into individual molds to set. Serve cold. Serves 2–4. Sprinkle fresh fruit on diet list—strawberries, raspberries, melon balls, etc.—with white wine. Let set until fruit has been penetrated. Then use as garnish for pudding.

Variation: Low-Calorie Peach Cream Delight—substitute 1 16-oz. can dietetic peaches plus the juice for the pears.

PURPLE HEART JELLO GRAND MARNIER

8 ripe plums
Artificial sweetener to taste
1-½ ozs. Grand Marnier (or
　cognac)

2 envelopes unflavored
　gelatin
½ tsp. orange extract
3 cups water

Slice plums coarsely. Add 3 cups water and sweetener. Stew plums on medium flame (on electric stove at medium) until barely tender. Add Grand Marnier and orange extract. Soften gelatin in 2 tbs. of cold water and add to preceding mixture. Pour into 1-quart mold or casserole dish. Place in refrigerator. Allow to chill until firm. For topping we recommend a Custard Sauce **. Serves 4.

RUM-CHOCOLATE PUDDING

1 envelope low-calorie
　chocolate pudding mix
1-½ cups milk

1 tbs. artificial rum or
　brandy
Artificial sweetener to taste

*** See Recipe Index*

Empty pudding mix into saucepan. Gradually stir in milk, and sweetener to taste. (We do not find low-calorie pudding mixes sweet enough and always add artificial sweetener. You may not feel this necessary.) Stir over heat until mixture starts to thicken. Before cooling add artificial brandy or rum. Pour mixture into individual dishes or mold. Refrigerate for 4 hours. Serves 4–6.

SHAMROCK JELLO RING

½ cup lime juice
1-½ cups water
1 tbs. unflavored gelatin
1 chicken bouillon cube
1 drop green food coloring

1 tbs. coarsely chopped
 parsley
Artificial sweetener equal to
 2 tbs. sugar

Sprinkle gelatin into water. Heat until dissolved. Add bouillon cube; stir until dissolved. Add the lime juice and sweetener and food coloring. Sprinkle the bottom of a 1-qt. mold with parsley. Spoon a little of the gelatin mixture over it and allow it to set. Then carefully pour the rest of the gelatin into the mold. Chill until firm. Serves 8–12.

SPICE STRIPS

½ cup melted shortening
1-¼ tsp. artificial liquid
 sweetener
2 eggs
1-⅓ cup gluten flour ***
⅔ cup soybean flour ***

2 tsp. baking powder
¾ tsp. ground cloves
1 tsp. cinnamon
½ tsp. nutmeg
½ cup water
¼ cup walnuts, chopped

Add liquid sweetener to melted shortening. Beat eggs; add to shortening. Mix and sift flour, baking powder and spices; add to egg mixture alternately with water. Spread in pan 15 x 10 x 1 inches. Sprinkle with walnuts. Bake in moderate 350-degree oven for 35 minutes. Cut into 36 pieces.

Printed with permission of Chicago Dietetic Supply, Inc.

*** *Buy in Health Food Store*

SOYBEAN GLUTEN SPICE CAKE

¾ cup gluten flour,
   sifted ***
¼ cup soy flour, sifted ***
1 tsp. artificial liquid
   sweetener
1 tsp. baking powder
3 tbs. corn oil

½ tsp. salt
1 tsp. cinnamon
½ tsp. nutmeg
¼ tsp. ginger
1 egg, beaten
½ cup water
2 tsp. vanilla

Sift dry ingredients together into a bowl. Mix liquid sweetener, corn oil, vanilla, beaten egg and water. Pour liquid into dry ingredients. Mix until smooth, but be careful not to overmix. corn oil, vanilla, beaten egg, and water. Pour liquid into dry Pour into greased loaf pan (approx. 8 inches by 4 inches). Bake at 350 degrees for 30 to 40 minutes, or until toothpick inserted comes out clean. Makes a small loaf 8 inches by 4 inches by 1 inch or can be baked as 6 cupcakes. Serves 6.

Printed with permission of Chicago Dietetic Supply, Inc.

If You Want to Compete with the Sundae Eaters, or You Are Serving a Blanc Mange or Mousse for Dessert, Make Yourself a:

STRAWBERRY FROU FROU

12 ozs. plain yogurt
12 ozs. chilled sugar-free
   strawberry soda
6–8 large strawberries
2 ozs. cold water

1 envelope unflavored
   gelatin
Artificial sweetener equal to
   ½ cup of sugar

Dissolve gelatin in cold water. Add artificial sweetener equal to ½ cup sugar. Place mixture in your blender. Add rest of ingredients and blend. When it starts to thicken, pour the contents of the blender into a deep Pyrex dish or into individual compote dishes and chill. Serves 6–8.

STRAWBERRY MOUSSE

2 cups fresh strawberries
2 envelopes unflavored
   gelatin

Artificial sweetener to taste
2 containers plain yogurt

*** *Buy in Health Food Store*

Chop strawberries in blender. Add yogurt and artificial sweetener. Dissolve gelatin in just enough boiling water and add to mixture. Put everything into blender and Blend or Whip for 60 seconds. Pour into individual dishes or into large casserole. Chill for 4 hours in refrigerator. Serves 6.

STRAWBERRY WHIP

2 envelopes unflavored gelatin	2 cups strawberries
2 tbs. cold water	1-½ cups water
1-½ tbs. unsweetened canned or fresh grapefruit juice	2 egg whites
	Artificial sweetener equal to ½ cup sugar

Dissolve gelatin in 2 tbs. cold water in mixing bowl. Add sweetener and grapefruit juice. Stir over heat until gelatin is completely dissolved. Stew berries in 1½ cups water and combine with gelatin mix. Stir well. Place mixture in refrigerator to chill and until it starts to thicken. Beat egg whites for 3 minutes or until peaks form. When mixture is beginning to thicken, fold in egg whites and pour mixture into individual glass compote dishes or 1-½-qt. ring mold. Chill for approximately 4 hours. Unmold onto platter. Fill center of ring with melon balls or any fruit you happen to have. Serve with ½ cup evaporated milk whipped with 1 tsp. artificially sweetened black cherry syrup, or our Brandy Sauce **. Serves 4.

TANGERINE AND ORANGE COMPOTE

3 navel oranges	1-½ oz. orange liqueur (artificial) ***
3 tangerines	
1 cup orange juice	Artificial sweetener equal to 1 tbs. sugar
1 tbs. orange rind	

Peel the fruit and remove the seeds. Slice the oranges thin lengthwise. Leave the tangerines in small segments. Place in layers in a fruit bowl. Bring the orange juice and rind to a boil, add the sweetener, and pour over the fruit. Place in refrigerator to chill. Pour the orange liqueur over fruit and serve. Serves 4–6.

** *See Recipe Index*
*** *Buy in Health Food Store*

ZABAGLIONE HG STYLE

For each person to be served use:
2 egg yolks
1 pkg. artificial sweetener
1 tbs. Marsala, kümmel or sherry

Beat the egg yolks and sweetener until pale and creamy. Add the Marsala or whatever liquor you use. Place in a double boiler over medium heat. Cook until it thickens. Serve either warm or cold in 4-oz. stem glasses.

Recipe Index

Acorn Squash
  with Applesauce, 112
  Baked, 113
  with Grapes, 113
  with Strawberries, 113
  Stuffed, 114
Almond-Stuffed Onions, 110
Apple and Cheese, 37
Apple Brown Betty HG, 132
Apple, Sharp Cheese and Soybean
    Balls, 33
Apricot
  Coffeecake, 132
  Delight Cake, 133
  Soufflé HG, 133
  Soup I, 51
  Soup II, 51
  Surprise, 54
Artichoke
  Bottoms and Chopped Veal, 104
  Flour Shells HG Style, 105
  Hollandaise, 104
  and Mushrooms, 104
  Salad, 54
  in White Wine, 105
Asparagus
  and Almonds, 105
  Soup, 46
  Tips Vinaigrette, 106
Aspic Salad, Luncheon, 58
Avocado
  Dressing, 123
  Salad Dressing, 123

Bacon, 66
Baked Custard, 143
Baked Fresh Tongue, 73
Baked Nectarines, 148
Baked Party Steak, 71
Baked Peaches, 148
Baked Veal Chops, 83
Barbecue Sauce, 123
Barbecued Broilers, 66
Barbecued Halibut Steaks, 93
Barbecued Spareribs, 71
Beef Bouillon
  Jellied, 46
  Snack, 38
Beef Roulades, 66
Bing Bang Jello, 139
Black Cherry Sauce, 125
Black-eyed Snapper, 101
Blackberry
  Grand Marnier, 134
  Ice, 134
  Mousse, 136
  Muffins, 136
  Sponge, 135
  Supreme, 135
Blue Cheese Salad Dressing, 124
Blueberry
  Bread-Cake, 39
  Midnight Pudding, 137
  Mousse, 136
  Muffins, 40
  Oat Cookies, 136
  Pudding, 137

Recipe Index

Blueberry *(cont.)*
  Snowball, 137
  Whip, Mock, 137
Boiled Salmon with
    Peppercorns, 97
Brandy Topping, 124
Bread, True HG, 45
Breaded Veal Cutlet, 83
Breakfast Menus, 7-15
Broccoli and Shrimp
    Casserole, 118
Broiled Butterfly Shrimps, 101
Broiled Grapefruit, 146
Broiled Haddock, 93
Broiled Lobster, 97
Broilers with Grapes, 73
Brown 'n Bake Chicken, 73

Caribbean Custard, 144
Carob Mousse, 138
Carrot and Orange Ring, 106
Cauliflower with Rice Wafer
    Sauce, 107
Cauliflowerssoise, 47
Caviar Spread, 124
Celery, Stuffed, 37
Chesse, Apple and, 37
Cheese Soufflé, 63
Cheesecake, 138
  HG Chocolate, 138
Cherry Soup, 51
Chicken
  Breasts, Stuffed, 76
  Brown'n Bake, 73
  and Frankfurter Salad, 55
  Fricassee, 74
  with Ham and Swiss, 75
  Herb Casserole, 118
  and Olive Mousse, 75
  Oriental, 76
  Ring, Jellied, 55
  Salad, 54
  and Shrimp, 76
  Stuffing, 76
Chocolate Bavarian, 140
Cinnamon Cookies, 141
Coconut Puffs, 141
Coffee
  Jello, Decaffeinated, 142
  Maple Jello, Decaffeinated, 141
Cold Cucumber Soup, 47

Cold Fresh Ham, 77
Cold Veal Salad, 61
Consommé, Jellied, 48
Corned Beef, 67
Cornish Hen and Frankfurter
    Salad, 55
Cottage Cheese
  Caraway Salad, 56
  and Fruit Salad, 56
Country Chicks, 84
Cranberry
  Bread, 40
  Crisp Mold, 125
  Crumble, 142
  Mold, Tangy, 56
  Muffins, 40
  Sherbet, 143
Cranshaw Melon,
    Fruit-Stuffed, 148
Cream Sauce, 126
Crema di Bagnomaria
  HG Style, 143
Creamed Veal, 84
Crepes Suzette HG Style, 139
Crumb Topping, 126
Cucumber Soup, 48
  Cold, 47
Curried Hake, 93
Custard
  Baked, 143
  Caribbean, 144
  Maple, HG Style, 147
  Sauce, 126

Date Coffeecake, 132
Decaffeinated Coffee Jello, 142
Decaffeinated Coffee-Maple
    Jello, 141
Demi Peanut Butter and Bacon
    Sandwich, 35
Deviled Eggs with Mustard, 34
Deviled Halibut Steaks, 94
Dill Sauce, 127
Dinner Menus, 22-32
Duck, Roast, 77

Easy Steak Dinner, 72
Egg Rolls, Miniature Chinese, 33
Eggplant
  Pancakes, 107
  with Dill, 107

Panned, 109
Red-Cap, 109
Soufflé, 108
Endive Fromage, 108
Energy Milkshake, 34

Filet of Sole
  in Dill Sauce, 102
  Fried, HG Style, 102
  Meuniere, 102
  with White Grapes, 103
Frankfurter Salad
  Chicken and, 55
  Cornish Hen and, 55
French Toast, Mock, 41
Fresh Bing Cherry and Port Wine
  Mold, 125
Fresh Salmon Chablis, 98
Fried Filet of Sole HG Style, 102
Fried Potatoes HG Style, 111
Frozen Raspberry Topping, 130
Fruit Cream Quickie, 145
Fruit Ring, 145
Fruit Salad
  Cottage Cheese and, 56
  Dressing, 127
  Plate, 57
Fruit-Stuffed Cranshaw
  Melon, 148

Gelatin Cheese Torte Pie
  Filling, 139
Gluten and Soy
  Biscuits, 41
  Bread, 42
Gluten Soybean
  Muffiins, 42
  Yeast Bread, 43
Gluten-Oat Bread, 41
Granual Meatloaf, 68
Grape and White Wine Sauce, 127
Grapefruit, Broiled, 146
Green Bean Parmesan Salad, 57
Green Melon Soup, Orange
  and, 52
Green Peppers, Stuffed, 86
Ground Ham and Pineapple, 79
Guacamole, 128

Haddock, Broiled, 93
Hake, Curried, 93

Halibut
  with Dill, 94
  Mousse, 94
  with Mustard Sauce, 95
  with Peanuts, 95
  Ring, 96
  Salad, 57
  Steaks
    Barbecued, 93
    with Curry Sauce, 96
    Deviled, 94
Ham
  and Chicken in Wine, 79
  Cold Fresh, 77
  and Corned Beef in Wine, 79
  Cured in Cider, 78
  Deviled, and Cheese Gelatin, 78
  Dip, 128
  Ground, and Pineapple, 79
  Mushrooms and, 79
  and Noodle Casserole, 119
  Roast Fresh, 80
  Stuffed Slices, 80
  and Veal Cutlets in Wine, 79
Ham-Cheese Balls, 34
Hash, Quick, 67
Hearts of Palm Salad, 60
HG Apricot Soufflé, 133
HG Chocolate Cheesecake, 138
HG Seafood Sauce, 130
Hollandaise Sauce, 128
  Mock, 128
Hot Dogs with Artichoke
  Shells, 67

Instant Cranberry Sauce, 126

Jellied Beef Bouillon, 46
Jellied Chicken Ring, 55
Jellied Consommé, 48
Jellied Tomato Soup, 50
Jello
  Bing Bang, 139
  Decaffeinated Coffee, 142
  Decaffeinated Coffee-Maple, 141
  Grand Marnier, Purple
    Heart, 150
  Key Lime Chiffon, 146
  Ring, Shamrock, 151

Key Lime Chiffon Jello, 146
Kosher Fry Beef, 66

Recipe Index

Lamb
  Ragout of, 81
  Shish Kebab, 81
Leftover Roast Veal Goulash, 85
Leftover Salad, 58
Lemon Pudding, 146
Lime Mold, 58
Lobster
  Broiled, 97
  Spicy, 97
Low-Calorie Pear Cream
  Delight, 150
Lunch Menus, 16-21
Luncheon Aspic Salad, 58

Macaroni Shells and Cheese, 119
Maple Custard HG Style, 147
Maple Delight, 147
Meatloaf, Granual, 68
Melon Balls Crème de Menthe, 148
Meringue, 129
Midnight Pudding, 137
Milkshake, Energy, 34
Miniature Chinese Egg Rolls, 33
Mixed Grill, 81
Mock Blueberry Whip, 137
Mock French Toast, 41
Mock Vichyssoise, 50
Mock Whipped Cream Sauce, 131
Mushroom Sauce, 129
Mushroom Soup Pureé, 48
Mushroom-Spinach Salad, 59
Mushrooms
  in Cream Sauce, 109
  and Sour Cream, 110

Nectarine Soup, 53
Noodle and Beef Casserole, 120
Noodle Mousse, 120

Onions, Almond-Stuffed, 110
Orange and Green Melon
  Soup, 52
Orange Compote, Tangerine
  and, 153
Orange-Bean Mold, 59
Our HG Salad Dressing, 129
Our Pepper-Pot Salad
  Dressing, 129

Panned Eggplant, 109
Peach
  Baked, 148
  Burgundy, 149
  Cake, 149
  Mumbo-Jumbo, 149
Peanut Butter
  and Bacon Sandwich, Demi, 35
  Biscuits, 43
  with Chopped Apple, 34
  Nut Balls, 35
Peanut Meatballs, 35
Peanut Veal Balls, 36
Pear Cream Delight,
  Low-Calorie, 150
Pears, Stuffed, 60
Pepburger, 68
Pepper Steak, 69
Peppers, Sautéed, 110
Pineapple, Chicken, and
  Spaghetti Casserole, 121
Pink Melon Soup, 52
Plum
  Muffins, 44
  Soup, 53
Poached Eggs à la Cheddar, 63
Pork Casserole, 121
Pork Chops
  and Cheese, 82
  with Olives, 82
  and Sour Cream, 83
Pot Roast
  Sparkling, 69
  Sweet and Sour, 70
Potage Asperges, 46
  à la Crème, 46
Potatoes, Fried, HG Style, 111

Quick Hash, 67
Quick Snacks, 37
Quick Spinach Soup, 49

Ragout of Lamb, 81
Raspberry
  Cottage Cheese Topping, 130
  Muffins, 44
  Oat Cookies, 136
  Omelet, 64
  Soda HG, 36
  Topping, Frozen, 130
Red Cold Salad, 60

Red-Cap Eggplant, 109
Roast Beef and Mustard, 70
Roast Duck, 77
Roast Fresh Ham, 80
Rum-Chocolate Pudding, 150

Salad Dressing
  Our HG, 129
  Our Pepper Pot, 129
Salmon
  Chablis, Fresh, 98
  with Peppercorns, Boiled, 97
  avec Poissonade au Charbon de
    Bois, 98
  Ring, 99
  Salad HG Style, 61
  and Soybeans, 99
  Steaks with Mixed Fruit, 100
  au Tarragon, 100
Salmon Caviar with Shallots, 124
Saumon au Tarragon, 100
Saumon avec Poissonade au
    Charbon de Bois, 98
Sautéed Peppers, 110
Seafood Newburg, 101
Shamrock Jello Ring, 151
Sherry-Mushroom Sauce, 131
Shish Kebab of Beef, 70
Shrimp
  Butterfly, Broiled, 101
  Omelet, 64
  Tidbits, 37
Snapper, Black-eyed, 101
Soup with Beef and Vegetables, 46
Soy and Beef Burger, 71
Soy Bread Loaf, 44
Soybean Gluten Spice Cake, 152
Spareribs, Barbecued, 71
Sparkling Pot Roast, 69
Spice Strips, 151
Spicy Broiled Lobster, 97
Spinach
  Custard, 111
  Delight, 111
  Omelet, 64
  Ring I, 112
  Ring II, 112
  Soup, 49
    Quick, 49
Springtime Vegetable Platter, 116

Squash
  Pancakes; Yellow, 114
  Pudding, 114
  Soup, 49
Steak
  Dinner, Easy, 72
  and Herbs with Mushrooms, 72
  Party, Baked, 71
Strawberry
  Frou Frou, 152
  Mousse, 152
  Muffins, 45
  Whip, 153
Stuffed Baked Tomatoes, 115
Stuffed Celery, 37
Stuffed Chicken Breasts, 76
Stuffed Green Peppers, 86
Stuffed Ham Slices, 80
Stuffed Pears, 60
Stuffing, 76
Sugarless Chiffon Cake, 140

Tangerine and Orange
  Compote, 153
Tangy Cranberry Mold, 56
Tomato Soup
  Jellied, 50
  à l'Orange, 50
Tomatoes, Stuffed Baked, 115
Tongue, Baked Fresh, 73
Tossed Salad, 61
True HG Bread, 45
Tuna and Cashew Casserole, 122
Tuna Ring, 103
Turnips
  Baked, 115
  Fried, 115

Veal
  and Almonds, 86
  Birds, 86
  and Chestnut Casserole, 122
  Chops
    Baked, 83
    and Cheese, 87
  Creamed, 84
  Cutlets
    Breaded, 83
    with Eggplant, 87
    au Vin, 87
  with Eggs, 89

Veal *(cont.)*
Fricandeau, 88
Goulash, Roast, Leftover, 85
Marsala, 89
and Mushrooms, 89
Roast I, 89
Roast II, 90
Salad, Cold, 61
with Salmon, 90
Scallopine with Sherry, 90
Shish Kebab of, 85
Stew, 91
Stuffed Zucchini, 91
Wiener Schnitzel, 92
Vichyssoise, Mock, 50

Waldorf Salad, 62

Watercress
Plus Dressing, 131
Soup, 49
Whipped Cream Sauce, Mock, 131
Wiener Schnitzel, 92

Yellow Squash Pancakes, 114
Yogurt
with Fruit, 38
Mix Sauce, 131

Zabaglione HG Style, 154
Zucchini
Casserole, 116
Omelet, 65
Pancakes, 116
Parmesan, 117
Stuffed, 117